Are You Gregg's Mother?

Charlotte G. Morgan

Legacy Book Press LLC
Davenport, Iowa

ACKNOWLEDGMENTS

Are You Gregg's Mother? has evolved over years of experience and reflection. Colleagues have read the manuscript and encouraged me to get it out into the world to hold a mirror up for other families, especially mothers, who are raising a child with mental illness. Those excellent mental health professionals who strive to help are invaluable resources and well worth the effort to find and consult. Clinical psychologist Susan Saandholland read the manuscript-in-progress and encouraged me to tell my story.

Nimrod Hall in Bath County, Virginia has been my summer writing retreat for three decades. There, former proprietor Frankie Apistolas supported my endeavors and listened, an invaluable sounding board. My writing colleague and mentor Cathryn Hankla heard these stories for years, as well, and gave support and advice.

In recent years, my regular writing community has narrowed to three women: Laura Gabel-Hartman, Jane Goette, and Mindy Quigley. All three have read this manuscript and found it deserving of a wider audience. I am ever grateful for their wise input.

My gratitude and acknowledgment would be incomplete without thanking and honoring my husband John and my son Gregg. Both believed in my ability to tell this story with honesty.

"The Letter" was originally published in the chapbook *TimeTravel* by Finishing Line Press in 2020.

DEDICATION

For Mothers

"Grown don't mean nothing to a mother. A child is a child. They get bigger, older, but grown. In my heart, it don't mean a thing."
~Toni Morrison

For the National Alliance on Mental Illness to which ten percent of the profits from the sale of this book will be donated.

CONTENTS

PROLOGUE

Gregg's daycare graduation occurred one bright June afternoon. Parents were invited to see the little ones get their "diplomas" and have cookies and juice afterward. We were outside, the sun was shining but not too hot, and I had a sense that things would work out for our broken family, eventually, even though I had no idea how. After the brief ceremony, I stood by myself while Gregg horsed around with some of his friends. He didn't hang on me much anymore, which pleased me. My ex-husband Will was standing off by himself, but that wasn't unusual.

One of the aides, a woman I'd seen often but hadn't officially met, walked up to me.

"Are you Gregg's mother?" she asked.

"Why yes, I am," I answered, smiling.

"Could I talk to you for just a moment? About Gregg?"

"Sure." We stepped away from the noisy children.

"I feel like I have to say this. I hope you won't be upset. But I need to tell you: Gregg's an angry little boy."

"What?" I lost my breath.

"I just thought you ought to know."

She walked away, leaving me with the sensation that I'd had the wind knocked out of me. I wanted to say, "Wait, what do you mean? Why would you say a thing like this?" But I couldn't speak. Gregg never threw tantrums, never hit other children or took their toys, never complained. A sweet-natured child, he hardly cried, unless he was physically hurt. Usually, there had to be blood for him to so much as a whimper. He was dear to me, petting my cheek, kissing me goodnight, telling me he loved me. I didn't know what to make of what this woman said. Except it hit a raw nerve.

I went up and hugged him goodbye—he was going with his dad for the weekend—and he had an innocent smile on his face, his cheeks all pink from playing. He looked like the most normal, healthy, happy boy in the world. But when I got in my car, I cried and cried.

She had to have him confused with someone else. Did she say Gregg? Certainly she meant some other boy.

Then why was I sobbing?

CHAPTER 1 -- SOME BABIES

"Some babies don't want to be born," my o.b. said, stretching a tape measure over my pregnant girth. He called out some numbers to the nurse, who was writing information in my chart.

Neither one looked at me. My mouth was dry. I needed to ask what that meant, don't want to be born, but I didn't. His answer couldn't be good. And this pregnancy had me on the verge of crying at any moment for no reason, my throat always tight, my voice shaky.

"Let's take a look inside." With that, he tapped my knee nearest him. He announced more numbers as his hand pushed up inside me. It didn't hurt. I was way past that. I was sure he must be checking the baby's skull, or my membranes. I was big on medical shows, like *Dr. Kildare* or *Ben Casey*, and liked to read anything that had to do with illness and health care. I told myself this was all routine, a regular part of every prenatal exam.

"Let me help you up." He peeled off his gloves, dropped them in a wastebasket, and pulled a rolling stool up by my head. Taking my upper arm, he steered as I grunted to an upright position and then looked over at him, curious. His smile was less than natural.

"I thought you had the dates wrong, Mrs. Smith. But turns out that's not the case."

"Right. Like I said, I'm certain about when I got pregnant. I told you that all along."

He shrugged, shook his head yes. "We got the results from the urine collection. This baby is what we call post-term."

I nodded, puzzled; in my obsessive reading about pregnancy, that was a description I'd missed. How bad could it be for the baby to grow a few extra weeks, though?

"So, let's see, the original estimated delivery date was"—the nurse handed him the open chart, pointed to a spot—"uh-huh, September 3. And it's"—he looked at his watch, "September 28th." He didn't say anything right away. I waited. "Baby's not gaining weight. Fact is, it seems to be losing. And it's not down in the canal at all, still pretty high. No cervical dilation." He stared at the chart some more, his eyes moving back and forth. "Tell you what, if you don't have the baby over the weekend, we'll put you in Monday morning and induce."

I nodded okay.

"Like I said, some babies get too cozy inside Mama, and they need a little help. All right?"

"Sure."

"Have your bag packed. I won't be on call this weekend,"—he headed for the door, the nurse close behind—"but you know Dr. S., you'll be in good hands."

I nodded. I preferred Dr. S., actually.

"Oh, and on your way out, tell the receptionist to schedule the hospital for early Monday, just in case. I'll put a note on the chart. And keep taking your prenatal vitamins." Reassuring smile, and he'd gone.

I sat there dumbfounded. I didn't have any idea if I should worry or not, but I tended towards worrying. I was too tired to even think of going to the library to look up post-term fetus. Scooting off the table, my hand holding onto my tight pregnancy ball, I stood, got my balance, and started to dress. If it had been any big deal, he would've alerted me, right? Of course. But then when Melanie was born, I hadn't even known that Will and I were Rh incompatible until after the delivery, when the doctor came around to explain the new shot I could sign for that would prevent that particular kind of blood problem in future babies. Blood problem? I'd realized, then, that I had to know the right questions to ask or I'd be a maternity ignoramus. I'd promised myself I'd be more assertive with the doctors the next time, but this baby-not-wanting-to-be-born thing had caught me off guard. I'd sat there like a pet rock and didn't ask one question. Well into my tenth month of pregnancy, I was tired all the time, lackluster, anxious for it to be over. All I could think of was going home and taking a nap.

Late Sunday night my labor pains started, sharp and hard, three minutes apart. Will took Melanie over to my girlfriend Carmen's apartment while I waited outside our place, leaning on the porch railing for support. My water hadn't broken—it had with my first—but the labor pains were regular and long. Three minutes apart. I knew it was time to get to the Emergency Room. I was relieved the baby had decided on his own to be born.

When we pulled up, an orderly wheeled out a wheelchair and whisked me into an examination room.

"The pains are really bad," I told the nurse when she told me to "hop up on the table."

She gave me a dubious look, said, "Lie down, Sugar, and let's take a look. We don't like to wake up the doctor too soon." After she moseyed over to put on a glove and strolled back to check me, her attitude changed. "Six centimeters. Let's see if Dr. S. is still in the hospital. You wait right here, Sweetie. I'll send someone in." Another pain hit, and I curled up and groaned, thinking I couldn't stand it. Still, I was so glad this was happening, so I wouldn't have to be induced. I'd read scary things about that, like too much pressure on the baby too fast.

Another orderly came with a bed, moved me onto it, and wheeled me to the o.b. area. *Things are gonna move fast now*, I thought. With Melanie, I'd labored six hours, and word had it that you could divide that by two for the second. So I could hope for a baby—a son, I knew, in my psychic way—by around three in the morning. That comforted me just long enough to endure the next labor pain.

A different female nurse—this one, to all appearances, mute—came and took my vital signs, kept her hands on me through two contractions, and then scurried out. Will had planned to be with me for the delivery, but I hadn't seen him since he'd opened the car door. I labored on, the pains intensifying, until Dr. S. came in. He was my favorite in the practice. Hardly much bigger than I was, about five feet three, he had the disposition of a sweet mama's boy rather than a short-guy Napoleon. I'd hoped he'd be on call when I went into labor.

"So, Charlotte, may I take a look? Are you ready to have this baby?" He was smiling, reassuring, already scrubbing his hands.

"Uh-huh," I managed, fighting through a pain.

"Pretty bad, huh? Coming pretty close?"

I nodded, fell back to rest for the next one.

Dr. S. got a confused look on his face for a few seconds as he examined my uterus. He kept feeling around, concentrating. When another pain started, he just said, "Okay, go ahead,"—as if I could stop it—and kept on checking me.

"Your waters haven't ruptured. And the baby's face up." He said this matter-of-factly. "I was worried you were too far along for the epidural, but we've got time, I think. Let's do this. Let's get the anesthesiologist in here to give you your shot." He looked like he wanted me to concur, so I nodded. "And once you're comfortable, I'll come back and break your bag of waters.

And then we'll see if your labor speeds up on its own. Is that okay with you?"

"Sure. But what about him being face up?"

He patted my arm. "Real often they turn on their own. Let's see if we can move him along after the membranes are ruptured, let mother nature take her course."

I didn't see him leave the room; I'd squeezed my eyes closed for another whammo of a pain.

The male anesthesiologist was taciturn, too, like the nurse, of the type that gave crisp orders and nothing more. "You will turn over on your side, please." I did. "This will be cold." I curled up. He waited. "You must be still now." I held my breath. "This will hurt a bit, then nothing." Afraid I might move, I froze. The needle going in did hurt, but I figured, anything to speed this up, get this baby out, even if I bite through my lower lip. "So, lie back, stay still. You will be comfortable in a few minutes. I will sit here."

I closed my eyes, as ill-at-ease as I had been all night. In a few minutes, I felt intense pressure in my back, like someone had dropped a cement block on me. "Ugh," I must've groaned, for he asked, "Something wrong?"

My face flushed, it hurt so badly. A different hurt, as if I were under a landslide, only the tons of mud had landed right over my lower back.

"My back," I murmured.

"Oh. Back pressure. Epidural cannot alleviate back pressure." He took my pulse and left. For the first time that night, tears pressed up from my eyelids. I didn't remember anything this overpowering from my first labor, though I'd had no medication at all until right when the baby was born—laughing gas. But no excruciating back pain.

Dr. S. came back into the room with a metal needle-like object about as long as a ruler—perhaps a bit longer. "Feeling better?"

"My back," I moaned.

He stood close to my head. "I'm sorry. Epidural works for labor pains. You won't feel those. But it can't do a thing for women in back labor. The pressure doesn't respond."

I didn't know what to say, except "At least it won't last long though, right?"

"I want to rupture the membranes now. My bet is things move along pretty quickly after that."

I only nodded. The pains had been predictable; I'd gotten to rest between them. But this back pressure was relentless. I felt like some cruel giant's fist was pushing down on my spine, and every nerve in that region was being twisted and crushed.

"Okay, Charlotte, this won't hurt at all," he said as he moved to the foot of the bed. "But you're going to need to stay perfectly still. This is extremely sharp, and we don't want it anywhere near the baby."

I opened my legs, braced myself.

"You ready? I'm going to do this now."

He was right, I didn't feel a thing. In no more than a second fluid came rushing out, as though a pitcher of warm water were pouring between my thighs. I was so relieved. Now the baby would come.

"Terrific. Let's get the nurse in here to clean you up. Daddy's been asking if he could see you." His kind face convinced me that things were normal now, and my son would be here any time.

Despite the pain, I smiled. I could endure this for half an hour, even forty-five minutes. By then I would've been laboring for about three hours. I could last. In a few more minutes I'd have my baby boy.

An hour and a half later I was lying in sweat, still not in the delivery room. Will must've come and gone; I couldn't remember. Dr. S. was talking about his childhood, something about not minding being small as a boy, and I could barely concentrate on what he was saying. He was trying to relax me. He was going to do another pelvic exam to see how the baby was progressing. The last time, about forty-five minutes before, the baby was still face up, still not engaged in the birth canal, and I was still only seven centimeters dilated. I remembered that.

"Okay, let's see if this stubborn little cuss is on its way."

Again he looked somewhat puzzled, none too pleased. "You've stopped dilating. And the baby hasn't moved since last time." He walked up to my head. "Let's try Pitocin, okay?"

I vaguely remembered reading about Pitocin. Wasn't it used to induce labor? Wasn't I already in labor? With this epidural, all I could feel was my traumatized backbone. I didn't know if I was still having labor pains or not. "It won't hurt the baby? Will it?"

"Of course not. It just might move things along a bit, intensify those labor pains. But you shouldn't feel it at all."

The anesthesiologist came back and put more medicine in the port, this time barely speaking. I didn't care; this labor was defeating me.

Another nurse came in and put an I.V. in my arm. Then she had me open my mouth and placed a tablet between my gum and my lip. Which was the Pitocin, the I.V. or the tablet? I had no idea. I felt too overwhelmed to fight the pain, too weak to even cry. I kept my eyes closed, only hoping for some comfort in the dark behind my eyes.

I know the nurse checked me at least one more time, and the doctor checked me at least once more, too, but mostly I was alone. I was way past chitchat, barely acknowledging their presence, only answering if I had to. Yes, my back hurt. Yes, I felt nauseous. Yes, I would agree to forceps. Forceps? I was groggy, but not too groggy to keep me from being scared.

The doctor was explaining that the baby had never turned; he was still "sunny side up," which was impeding his ability to push through the birth canal. We should try forceps. Try?

I was wheeled to the delivery room. I was awake, but beyond any capability of helping with the birth. Will was there, in green scrubs and a mask, his face stolid.

A nurse told him, "If you feel like you're going to throw up or faint, get out of the way; we'll walk over you." His eyes looked scared. I wondered what the doctor had told him, but I didn't want to know.

Someone propped my feet in the stirrups. I could see my legs trembling. It was a strange sight, seeing my legs look like they were having a seizure, but having no physical sensation of it. The doctor was pressing down on the baby with one hand, his other up inside me. He stood and must have indicated he wanted something, because a nurse handed him a set of forceps. I had never seen any—the word was bad enough. They looked like gigantic tongs, about the size of an old-fashioned rug beater. Like some torture tool from that old *SNL* skit, "Theodoric of York". He must have tried to turn the baby. I was watching, but that part of myself was under a green cloth tent, so I couldn't see a thing. Or feel anything except my back.

When he stood, he still had the forceps in his hand. He gave them back to the nurse, and a different nurse brought him another set, only larger. I thought, *A vet could deliver a foal with those.*

"Okay, come on this time," he said as he bent over me, and sure enough, within a couple of minutes, he handed over the forceps and reached to turn my son and pull him into the breathing world.

A nurse took him right away, and the doctor smiled. "You were right, he's a boy. He looks fine." Will came over and took my hand. I collapsed against the bed, too spent to even look. I saw the clock, though; it was 6:43 in the morning. This labor had been longer than Melanie's.

When someone handed me the swaddled baby, he looked like a little old man with bruises on his forehead. His skin was peeling, like from a bad case of sunburn. His scrunched face was none too happy, though he wasn't crying. "Hi, Gregg," I said, staring into his worried dark eyes. They seemed to say to me, "I was every bit as scared as you were, Mom." So our first shared emotion had been fear. The first second I'd held Melanie, I'd felt a letdown of some new overpoweringly amazing sensation, like the letdown of my milk. Without a doubt, it was maternal love, a powerful sense of knowing "real" love for the first time. With Gregg, I only felt a rush of relief.

I handed him to his father and closed my eyes, glad he had ten fingers and ten toes, unable to stay awake a second longer. I was so exhausted I forgot to ask his Apgar score.

The next time I opened my eyes I was alone in a hallway, on the same rolling hospital bed. A baby's screams had jangled me out of deep sleep, and somehow I knew that it was MY baby crying. Not hungry crying, not fussy crying, screaming. In pain. A nurse came to check on me. I had to lie flat for another eight hours, something about the epidural. They were waiting for a room in maternity; my baby was being circumcised. Both of us should be "upstairs" on the ward in no time. The baby's shrieks were pitiful. I hated myself for signing the permission papers. I fell back to sleep.

The rest of my hospital stay comes through in that paradoxical hazy clearness of a dream. In my room, I was fretful. My o.b. came in. Despite the fact that I was a jumble of nerves, he assured me I was fine. My episiotomy was clean— no tearing. No excess bleeding. Was I having headaches? The epidural sometimes causes headaches. No— I couldn't stay awake long enough to know if I was having headaches. Good. If I had them I'd know it. I needed my rest. I wanted to breastfeed. Of course; they'd probably bring the baby next feeding. He really wasn't involved in that. Talk to the nurse or the pediatrician.

When he left I felt beyond alone. I guess it was too early for my husband to visit. He'd stayed, I was told, until I was safely in my room and Gregg was in the nursery. He had to be exhausted, too. But more than anything I wanted to hold the baby, to see him again now that I was half-awake. Alert only meant jittery, though. My legs were still trembling. The maternity ward was abuzz, so there was no way I'd get back to sleep, even though I could barely turn my head from side to side.

The pediatrician came by; the baby was eating well. What? Eating what? We were breastfeeding. They'd fed him in the nursery so I could rest. He showed no signs of birth trauma, except for the bruising. I'd forgotten about the bruising. It should go away in a couple of days, no problem. His Apgar? Nine. He was six pounds seven ounces, eighteen inches. That was all? He'd felt enormous. No, he'd probably lost a few ounces during the past four weeks. He was definitely post-term, had all the signs: rough skin, especially on elbows and knees, low birth weight—though still within the normal range. Should I be worried? This I remember with clarity: "Mrs. Smith, please: we'll let you know when it's time to worry."

When a nurse finally brought him to me that first morning, he was in an isolette, sucking a pacifier. The woman handed me a swab of some sort and ordered me to clean my nipples. I'd nursed Melanie, I wasn't a rookie, but I did as I was told, noticing that the gauze smelled like those towelettes waitresses hand out at barbecue restaurants. Surely I wasn't wiping my nipples with alcohol? I didn't care, though. I was anxious to hold my baby and feed him and have some semblance of normalcy settle over us. Enormous hard breasts exposed, I held out my arms, said, "Okay," and she picked Gregg up, wrapped him tightly, clucking over him, and handed him over. I met her eyes, said, "I'd prefer you not give him a pacifier, please," and she glared at me as she pushed the cart out of my room.

Gregg's face was far calmer, and he latched onto my nipple with ease, sucking naturally. His eyes stared into mine, and I swear he looked as relieved as I felt. For a quiet half-hour, we held onto one another and the world was right. He was nobody's pretty thing, as my grandmother would've said, with those squished-in bruises on his forehead and that sallow skin, but he was going to be fine. The doctor had said so.

After they took him away, a different nurse came in and told me it was time for my sitz bath. Couldn't I take a shower? No—still too early after my epidural. She had me sit in a pan of warm water, told me she'd be back in about a half an hour. It did feel soothing, at first, but then as it cooled, I was uncomfortable. My back hurt. When she finally came back around, she brought a fresh pan of clean hot water so I could wash my face and brush my teeth, assuring me that after lunch they'd have me up and around. Never the helpless type, I regretted that epidural more and more. No one had told me about the tremors or the headaches or the not being able to get up for eight hours. I didn't ask the right questions again.

Will came, all flowers and smiles. He'd seen Gregg through the nursery window. A nurse had held him up, and he thought the baby looked fine. He didn't say a thing about the bruises. I gave him both doctors' reports, and I could tell that in his taciturn way he was as delighted as only a new dad could be. He helped me put on a regular gown from my bag, gave me my lip gloss and a comb, and I perked up considerably, giving in to a sense of calm for the first time in over a month. He sat with me while I rested, and in a little while, a nurse poked her head in and told us he could walk me up and down the hall now, if I promised to hold onto his arm. When I stood, I was stunned at how weak my legs were, how much my butt hurt, but glad to be up.

We went to the nursery and found Gregg in the baby boy Smith isolette; he was sleeping, breathing easily, but a blue pacifier lay beside his head. They'd ignored me. I was peeved. I'd call the pediatrician's office. Pacifiers were not good for nursing babies.

Will left, both of us at ease. He'd work all afternoon, then come back for evening visiting hours. I'd rest, finally. No doubt we'd be able to take Gregg home in the morning.

The two o'clock feeding went just as smoothly as the morning one. Gregg had not cried at all, either time. He was a dear, calm baby. Afterward, I was so tired I decided I'd put off calling his doctor's office until after I'd had a nap. Three to five were the only quiet hours on the maternity ward, it appeared, and I needed the sleep.

As it turned out, the pediatrician called me around four. I woke from a deep, calm sleep to the phone ringing. I almost didn't answer but thought it might be my parents calling. They were keeping Melanie at our apartment, and I figured my four-year-old daughter wanted to talk to her mama about her new baby brother. But it was the doctor.

"We're sending Gregg upstairs, Mrs. Smith." Upstairs? That simple word sounded ominous.

"What do you mean?"

"To Neonatal Intensive Care."

"Why? You said he was fine."

"The nurses called about his color. He's jaundiced. We're going to have to treat that."

"What exactly does that mean?" I had a vague thought of liver problems.

"I'll stop by to see you after I finish with his papers. It's serious but treatable. We'll talk."

And he hung up. For the first time, I started crying uncontrollably, weeping so hard I couldn't remember Will's number at work. I couldn't get my head around it. I knew jaundice had something to do with the liver and blood, but I thought we'd fixed that with the shot after Melanie was born. Could there be some other cause? Was it something really bad? He'd said serious, but how serious? The entire pregnancy I'd worried about this baby, knew something "wasn't right." I cried until I was so exhausted I must've fallen asleep.

I woke up when an aide brought in a dinner tray. "Got you some supper." I jolted to a sitting position, grabbed the phone, and

14

dialed Will. As soon as I heard his voice I started weeping again, incoherent. I somehow got out the words jaundice and intensive care, and he hung up.

I didn't see the doctor; perhaps he came by when I was asleep. When Will got there, he rang for a nurse, but she wouldn't tell us anything other than that parents were allowed to visit NICU at any time; we didn't have to adhere to regular visiting hours. She walked us to the elevator and told us where to get off and turn.

When we got up there (upstairs), holding onto one another, the nurses were an entirely different tribe of human beings. Their faces shone with kindness and concern. They acted as if we were the only two parents they had to deal with. We sat down, and a nurse explained about jaundice as much as she could. It was a neonatal condition in a certain percentage of babies. Yes, it involved the blood and the liver. It meant for some reason the liver wasn't able to cleanse the blood. There were a variety of reasons. A neonatal specialist would have to examine Gregg. He would talk to us about his hunches and his prognosis. Until then we were welcome to see Gregg any time of day or night. We couldn't rock him—he would be in a bilirubin tank until the jaundice reversed or until he had a total blood exchange. The liver should start to function. No, I couldn't nurse him until the specialist agreed. My milk might have something to do with causation of the jaundice.

Her kindness unhinged me, and I sat there weeping silently. Will, blanched, didn't say a word. When I was able to stand, she helped us into sterile gowns and showed us how to clean our hands properly. By then I only wanted to grab my baby and run from that room and never come back, to take him to some primal place where there were no doctors or nurses or pacifiers and nurse him until he was well. But the very things my instincts told me to do were the things I couldn't.

The woman took us through the automatic door into the humming world of newborns in distress, walked us past babies the size of wallets to Gregg's isolette, and my knees buckled under

15

me. He had on a black mask covering his eyes, and a similar black band where a diaper should've been covering his genitals. Like some newborn criminal. Sucking a pacifier, he was under a set of lights that emphasized the sickly yellow color of his skin. I reached out and touched his skinny foot, noticing punctures on his heel.

"We have to take blood every hour, to be sure it's not getting any worse." I had to turn away, even though I wanted to stay, to kidnap my son.

Two days later, I had to leave the hospital without my baby boy. When we came back for him later that week, Will and I sat in the waiting room a couple of chairs apart, him thumbing through magazines, me ready to jump out of my skin. I sensed that our marriage was damaged. A strange disconnection had settled over us. The gap between his stoicism and my emotional needs was too wide.

And though it doesn't make medical sense, I am sure that Gregg, too, from his traumatic birth through his stay in ICU, was damaged, perhaps beyond repair. Only I didn't know for certain how for almost twenty years.

CHAPTER 2 -- THE BEST BABY

Gregg was "the best baby," as nursed babies often are. He didn't sleep, but he wasn't cranky or colicky. Melanie had slept through the night at two months old, but those first two months had been a sleepless blur, with her tucking up her chunky little legs and screaming for an hour after every feeding. Still, she'd gained so much weight so fast even her pediatrician had been surprised—nursing was not the preferred form of infant feeding in 1969 when she was born. The colic ended at eight weeks and she slept like a champ from then on. Gregg, who rarely cried, rarely slept as well. He wanted to eat every two hours, round the clock. He'd sleep for brief spells, then be awake, looking around, alert and still. Though taking care of him was exhausting, I couldn't complain. He was home and healthy.

Still physically and emotionally wrecked myself from my extended pregnancy and bizarre childbirth, it was all I could do to get through the days. Getting Melanie up in the morning, fed, dressed, and content playing; trying to catch a nap the few times Gregg slept for half-hour or hour stretches; taking care of him when he was awake; and bathing and reading to Melanie at bedtime should have been a cakewalk. But I was a mess. Too nervous to really rest but home with a baby who was relatively easy to care for, I was unwilling to call my jitters postpartum depression. I wasn't unhappy, I was just constantly worried and nervous. But I'd always been kinda anxious—the family complaint, as my Aunt Ella called it.

My attention to my marriage was nil, to such a degree that I wasn't even concerned about my non-relationship with Will. He was great with the children when he came home from work, he didn't push me in any way, and he was as patient as the day is long. That we barely talked was not an issue that showed up on my radar.

All my close friends, except for my new friend Carmen, were in Richmond, where I'd grown up. Carmen lived in the complex and came over for a little bit every day, often taking Melanie home to play with her older daughter Christine, but she had two children of her own to tend to and couldn't be much help with the new baby. My parents had left when I came home from the hospital, before Gregg even got out of NICU. They'd stayed with Melanie as long as I'd needed them, but they both had jobs, and neither was the help-out-in-a-crisis type. Nobody acted like this birth had been a crisis in the first place. When my girlfriend Julia Ann, who I'd known since junior high school, called and offered to come up to northern Virginia and help for a few days, I tried to say no but she wouldn't let me. When she arrived, I just sat on the sofa and nursed Gregg while she did everything from preparing food to washing windows.

The second day she was there she insisted that Will and I go out to dinner together that evening. Though she hadn't said a word to me about our relationship, I'm sure she saw our lack of intimacy and it concerned her. She'd been a psychology major in college, she knew me well, and nothing much got past her. We'd only be gone a couple of hours. After a feeding, Gregg was content to sit in his punkin seat as long as he was in the same room with someone, usually me. Only four, Melanie wouldn't be a problem for Julia Ann. She'd never been a whiner/clinger. I didn't much want to go, but my friend pushed us out the door.

Will and I went out to a swank candle-lit restaurant nearby, leaving Gregg with a bottle of expressed milk. I dolled up, he complimented, and we sat in that dim dining room, all forced smiles and stilted conversation.

"You look great in that dress; nobody could tell you had a baby two weeks ago." I nod. "Except for the gigantic boobs." I smile. "I don't mind those one bit." Much as I tried, I couldn't relax and flirt during that steak and wine dinner; being away from the baby didn't feel right. Deep down, I was still irrationally mad at Will. How could he have read a magazine while Gregg was in intensive care? How could he have been so detached, so calm?

When we got home, Julia Ann was walking the floor with Gregg, who was red-faced and screaming. He had pinpoint broken blood vessels all over his cheeks.

"He's been like this ever since you left. He wouldn't even take the bottle." Julia Ann, a mom herself, ever-unruffled, was clearly glad we were home. And so was Gregg. I grabbed him, sat down, opened my dress, and offered him my swollen breast. He began nursing right away, so fast he made those little gasps babies make sometimes when the milk's coming out too fast. I knew I shouldn't have gone, and neither Will nor Julia Ann argued with me. Melanie was on the sofa with a book, curled up against me, ignoring Gregg. It had not been a good evening. This baby wasn't ready to be away from his mother again yet. Both of us knew things weren't right.

We liked our two-bedroom condo in Fairfax; we'd converted the walk-in closet in our bedroom into Gregg's mini-nursery. I could easily put him down, go to bed, and hear him when he stirred for a feeding. Will slept like a brick—what could he do anyway? I often lay awake at night, listening to Gregg breathing, even when I was too exhausted to move, even as I wished that just for once he'd sleep for four hours. My mind wouldn't rest, though. Our closed-off apartment world suited me as I tried to manage my baby's needs and my daughter's demands and get a grip on my own anxieties.

My dear college friend Nancy lived outside Richmond on a hundred-plus acre farm with her husband Andy and their four-year-old son Matthew, born just a couple of months after Melanie. In her rural community, the families had extravagant Halloween celebrations, and she called to convince me to bring the baby and come for the holiday, on a weekend that year.

"Come on, Charlotte. Andy and Will can take Matthew and Melanie around trick-or-treating—the houses are far apart, and they'll stop for a beer at everybody's—and you and I can stay here and talk. You said the baby's no trouble." I loved Nancy like the sister I'd never had, my missing twin; visiting her would be a tonic. She was funny, no-nonsense, loving, and real. Plus she was a breast cancer survivor, and I knew I could talk to her about absolutely anything, including my non-functioning marriage. She'd find some positive spin. So we went, even though Gregg was only thirty days old. Melanie was thrilled. We dressed her like a gypsy, with lots of beads and bangles and a scarf covering her hair, and Nancy and I had a wonderful three hours yakking while we took turns rocking Gregg.

When Andy got back, after Melanie and Matthew had squealed off to his room with the loot, he asked if I'd noticed the big lump on Melanie's left jaw. "If she's got mumps I'm gonna kill you, Charlotte." What lump? How had I missed my daughter having a lump?

Nancy was unconcerned. "Come on, Andy; it's probably not mumps. And even if it is, it'd be good for Matthew to have them before he goes to school."

I was stymied. "What bump? Show me, Andy."

We called Melanie back, and sure enough, she had a lump the size of a hard-boiled egg along her left jawline. How had I missed it? As a former first-grade teacher, I had seen and felt mumps, though. I was remembering the swelling as fleshy feeling. This was hard.

"I don't think it's mumps, but I have no idea what it could be. I'll give the pediatrician a call in the morning." It wasn't like me to call a doctor on a Sunday morning, even though I was a worrywart, but this frightened me, that inside mom radar registering something bad. I told myself that everything was feeling scary to me these days, that ever since Gregg's "extra month" inside me, I'd been a wreck. While Will and Nancy and Andy assured me there was bound to be some simple solution, I fretted all night. Gregg, of course, kept me company.

Talking to my brilliant young pediatrician the next morning didn't help. I got the one on call, Dr. Schwartz, and he told me to come right back to Northern Virginia and he'd meet us at his office. He had some other emergency cases to see, anyway, and this did not sound like mumps to him. In any case, with a new baby in the house, he wanted to see Melanie that day.

When we got there, only one car was in the parking lot of this huge, busy practice—his, I guessed—and he let us into the office himself. I left Will and Gregg in the waiting room and went back into an examination room with Melanie, who was rumpled and disagreeable from too little sleep and too much candy. He took his time palpitating the lump on her jaw.

Immediately, he said, "This isn't mumps." And he felt all around that jawline and the other side as well. He asked me when I'd first noticed this growth. That word "growth" stupefied me. With all my curiosity about medical issues, I hadn't for a second thought about this thing on her face as a "growth." I had to admit to him that I hadn't noticed it at all, and neither had my husband. A friend had identified it just the night before. How had I been imperceptive with my daughter?

He had Melanie hop down from the table and said, "Let's go back out with Mr. Smith, so I can talk to you together." Taking

Melanie's hand, I felt as if I were about to get the blow I'd been flinching against for weeks—only I'd been sure it had to do with the baby.

Will stood when we came into the room; oddly, Gregg was sleeping. He seemed like no more than a bundled towel next to his six-foot, football-player-framed daddy.

"Please sit, Mr. Smith. Both of you, sit down."

I told Melanie to go find a book at the play table; she hesitated, but only for a second. I sat down beside Will.

"This growth on Melanie's jaw is disturbing. The possibilities, well, neither of them is something a parent wants to hear." He looked from one of us to the other. "I'm going to need you to bring her in for blood work first thing in the morning," he started writing an order on a prescription pad.

"What are you thinking, doctor? What exactly are you looking for?" I don't know how Will was able to say those words. My mouth muscles were cement.

"Could be a form of leukemia." He paused. "There's something else, pretty rare, I've studied with a professor over at Children's who's doing the research, but it's a long shot. I've never seen a case myself."

"What's that?" Will persisted.

"I probably shouldn't even mention it. It's called Atypical TB. It presents like this, but usually, there's bruising, I recall from my med school days."

Tuberculosis? Wasn't that curable? Would she have to go away? Would the baby get it too? Anything sounded better than leukemia, though.

Dr. Schwartz handed me the prescription form. "Like I said, come first thing. The lab's just down the breezeway from our offices. They'll be expecting you. We'll go from there."

"What time do they open? The lab?" Will asked.

"Technicians get here at 7:30. Knock on the door. Someone will let you in." He shook Will's hand, patted me on the shoulder. "And don't worry about the baby. Neither of these is contagious."

Don't worry about the baby? Those words echoed in my head. All I'd been doing was worrying about the baby. I'd been so afraid that something else was wrong with him that I'd missed something wrong with my daughter.

Somehow I picked up my purse, took Melanie's hand, and got into our car. I have no idea how. In 1973, newborn car seats weren't required or even much encouraged. I took the baby and started nursing him, in total opposition to my edict Never Wake A Sleeping Baby. To say I was a zombie on the drive to our apartment would be an exaggeration. I think Melanie slept the half-hour ride, exhausted by her Halloween visit with Matthew and also, I'm certain, by the Sunday morning visit to the doctor and the peculiar behavior of her parents. Will and I didn't try to talk. I didn't know what to say, and I'm certain neither of us wanted to break down in front of Melanie. She was our beautiful, perfect, super-bright girl. Sure, she'd had ear infection after ear infection the year before—so many that the doctors had recommended her having her tonsils out, an unusual decision at the time. She'd had that surgery in the spring while I was pregnant. But leukemia? Or TB? Such thoughts had never so much as crossed my worry-wart mind. I was way out of my anxiety league, and all I could do was nurse the baby and be still, trying to hold myself together.

Will unloaded the car, unpacked the bags, behaved like a caring husband and father the rest of the day. Melanie didn't take naps, but she didn't mind a quiet time reading in her room. A few months earlier she'd asked me to stop reading out loud to her, claiming, "I can read faster inside my head." Tired herself, she was content to prop up on her bed and silent read. After our lunch— Will made sandwiches—I put Gregg down, hoping for one of his hour naps, and Will and I stretched out on our bed and held one

23

another. Words weren't necessary. Both of us understood that this was way too big, and out of our control.

Will drove Melanie back to the doctor's early the next morning, negotiating the horrible Fairfax traffic while I stayed home with the baby. Then he brought her home and went to work; he had to work. I knew he couldn't hang around our apartment waiting for the doctor to call. I couldn't call anyone, either, couldn't say those horrible words out loud. The hours dragged, but I moved from one mommy job to the next, keeping both children right with me all morning.

Around one, Dr. Schwartz called. "It's not leukemia." That's all I needed to hear. "I've already called Dr. X at Children's Hospital. He's the national authority on pediatric Atypical TB; he's expecting to see you and your husband and Melanie in the morning at 9. He's on the 4th floor. I wouldn't take the baby."

Did I thank him? I'm not sure. I know I didn't ask any questions. When I called Will and got him on the line, I could barely say "Atypical TB." We decided to talk more that evening— neither of us had any idea what that diagnosis meant, but it wasn't leukemia, and we knew that could be deadly. At least we could allow ourselves to be hopeful now.

Carmen would come up to my place and bring Christy and her two-year-old Jenny; I'd express milk and leave it for Gregg, enough for at least three feedings. Carmen didn't hesitate to agree to keep him as long as it took. Any drive into D.C. required planning for delays, perhaps hours in traffic. They were building the Metro, and backups were the norm. We'd leave early, around seven.

Her girls could look at television—a rare treat at my house—and Carmen would be free to walk Gregg all morning. She was no novice where screaming babies were concerned; her first-born had been a handful. Gregg was a squirmer, still, when anyone held him except me, even his dad. I didn't need to tell her any of the things the baby would need, though, which was a good thing, because by that point I was practically non-communicative.

Everything was out of whack, and I was helpless to fix it. Here I was, leaving my newborn again, when I knew it was hard on him, hard on us both. But I had to go to the hospital with my four-year-old.

At the time, Children's Hospital was still in its old brick facility in mid D.C., and it was a scary/miraculous place. We found our way to Dr. X's office, and he will forever remain in my mind and heart as right-next-door to a saint. Greying, with an open, wise face, he called Melanie over to him right away, asked if he could look at her chin, commented on what a polite little girl she was. As he indicated for Will and me to sit, he chattered with her, making eye contact all the while. Somehow I relaxed a hair, feeling safer already, as if despite the unpredictable nature of the past month we'd landed in the exact right place.

Melanie on his knee, he turned to us. "Mr. and Mrs. Smith,"—he looked directly into our eyes—"we're all lucky Dr. Schwartz was such a brilliant pediatric resident here at Children's. I don't suspect many of his group remember my ten-minute talk on Atypical TB. And we're doubly lucky he's your pediatrician. You have a delightful daughter here, and Dick Schwartz is right on target: that's what she has, Atypical TB." Melanie climbed down and came to lean against me, keeping her attention on Dr. X. "I'm sure you've never heard of it, and I'm certain you have many questions." We nodded. "Would it be all right with you all if I have one of my assistants take Melanie to our playroom? I have a number of questions myself."

The upshot was, after over an hour's consultation, that Melanie had probably caught this dust-borne mycobacteria at Nags Head, on our annual family vacation. He'd need to check her blood, but from our description of her tonsillectomy and our visit to the coast mid-summer, the doctor said he could speculate that that had been the onset. As to the prognosis, she'd need surgery, no ifs, ands, or buts. As quickly as he could schedule it, with the best pediatric surgeon on staff. Without surgical removal, the infected area, which was in her lymph node, would grow until it exploded out of the side of her face. Surgery was unavoidable. Complicating things was the likelihood that an important nerve ganglia controlling that side of her face was involved—they wouldn't know for certain until they opened it, which would be intricate— and paralysis or partial paralysis of that side of the face could result. The lymph node would be removed, so the filter for germs on that side of her face would be gone permanently.

Dr. X never hurried his explanation and answered every one of our questions. He wanted to do skin-pops on her arm on that side to verify his analysis of where the germ originated, if we didn't mind. He'd insert the different strains, and the one to react over the next forty-eight hours would be "it." He was writing the medical text, the first of its kind on Atypical TB, and he'd appreciate our willingness to contribute. She'd be in the hospital for four to five days. One of us could stay with her at all times. We'd meet the surgeon and anesthesiologist ahead of time; they'd visit with us and Melanie. The sooner the better.

Melanie came back, happy and at ease, and he described what he wanted to do on her arm, writing inky letters and drawing circles and making little sticks, and she agreed without any sign of fear. He did about eight skin-pops, like those in allergy testing, and photographed her arm and jaw a number of times, and while she winced, she never so much as cried. He explained that he'd see her in a couple of days, that when she came back he'd take more pictures of her arm, that one of the places would bubble up, like a blister, but she wasn't to worry. He was going to take care of everything. As floored as I was by the seriousness of all this, I believed him.

It was only when we got to the car that I thought of Gregg for the first time that morning. I needed to nurse, but I'd have to endure the one-hour minimum drive home with my breasts brick-hard and leaking. What would we do with Gregg while Melanie had surgery and recuperated in the hospital? Babysitting that long was too much to ask of Carmen. How could I be at the hospital with Melanie and at home breastfeeding him? How would he deal with these separations? This was too fast and too complicated. Melanie was jabbery in the back seat, so I got control of myself and played word games and sang songs with her until we got back to the house.

Will made all the calls to our parents and the arrangements for his mother to be ready to come whenever we got the word that the surgery was scheduled. We'd barely gotten beyond the four weeks of waiting for Gregg to be born, and now we were telling them all that we had another child in medical crisis. It was too much too soon. Will's mother Margaret was a kind-hearted, dear woman, with one of those massive shelf-chests a person could rest her head on and sob. But we'd never been close. Will's younger sister didn't much like me, so there'd been a bit of distance between me and Margaret. She was a terrific grandmother, bringing Melanie darling clothes that were more expensive than we could afford at the time, finding everything her granddaughter did adorable. I knew she'd be wonderful with Gregg, but he was still so small, and so needy. Would he be too much for her? She was white-haired, in her late fifties, short of breath from overwork and possibly high blood pressure (she would never complain). Besides, she couldn't drive. How would she get here from Fredericksburg? What if she had an emergency with the baby? But Will took care of it all. And true to his word, Dr. X called that very afternoon with a time for us to check into the hospital: Melanie would come early Monday, only five days away. He'd been able to schedule the surgeon he wanted; she'd have her operation that Tuesday morning at 6:30 a.m. The surgeon would meet us and talk to us about the procedure Monday around 1:00, and they'd do her complete workup that day. Dr. Schwartz was sending over her records.

So it was real. Somehow the days passed. I'm not sure I left the house, even to walk the baby. We went back to the hospital that one time to have Dr. X read Melanie's skin pops; his hypothesis about Nags Head had been correct. He wrote on her arm some more and took more photographs. She would be in his medical text. He couldn't tell us much more about the surgery, only that we were in the best hands in the country for this type of complicated facial procedure.

We got through the weekend as though nothing were wrong. Gregg nursed often, slept little. I wondered what impact the separation and all the tension would have on him, but I couldn't linger on those thoughts. Melanie was about to have surgery. Will went for his mother on Sunday. Her good cheer and positive outlook were a welcome addition to our lives; we needed her. She loved being with Melanie, brought her all kinds of presents like coloring books and crayons and stickers.

And she'd only seen Gregg once, through the nursery window, so she was content to sit on the sofa with him nestled against her enormous chest, assuring me, "We'll be just fine together here. You needn't worry a bit." Since, mercifully, the baby didn't appear restless with her, I accepted her reassurance with gratitude. I had to. We all tried to go to bed early that night, but none of us slept much, except Melanie. For once I was glad Gregg wanted to eat often during the night. I'd be spending long days at the hospital, but I'd be home nights when Will slept in the room with Melanie, so I was hoping the baby wouldn't be too fussy about the bottle during the days. I hated to think of Margaret pacing the floor with him for hours. Her health wasn't that good. But mostly I hated to think of him, still so young and small, separated from his mother and the comforts of nursing for days at a stretch.

Will, Melanie, and I left early for the hospital. She acted happy about her little red plastic suitcase and new nightgowns and brand new hospital toys. If I'd thought it possible, I would've determined that Dr. X had hypnotized her. She showed no fear at all, even when we got to her room. The hallways on the surgical floor were painted from floor to ceiling with enormous colorful Mother Goose figures. The nurses dressed in flowered smocks instead of white uniforms—something new to me—and each one was sunnier than the last. When the surgeon came by—a tall, broad-shouldered youngish man with hands the size of pocketbooks, Dr. Altman—he shook Melanie's hand first. She thrived on all the attention and flitted around in her floor-length nightgown like one of Peter Pan's pals. When the doctor took us down to the lounge to talk, she was content playing alone.

The surgery would take at least three hours, probably longer. A lot depended on the nerve involvement. The rather large mass had begun to bruise, indicating that we'd gotten her treatment none too soon. He hoped he wouldn't need to damage any nerves removing the growth and the diseased lymph node; if it was unavoidable, there would be some paralysis on that side of her face. He'd do his best, but he wouldn't know specifics until he got inside. He'd try to let us know something as soon as possible, but once he opened her up, she would be his only concern. He wouldn't keep us waiting longer than was necessary. Healing would take time, but scarring would be minimal. She probably wouldn't require plastic surgery.

This kept getting bigger, growing darker like the tumor on Melanie's jaw. I couldn't be much comfort to Will, nor him to me. His stoicism was a blessing that day. I don't think I could've smiled for another person except Melanie. When we got back to her room, she showed off a handmade sock doll one of the nurses had brought her. While the young woman explained her surgery to her, she'd drawn a mark on the doll's chin where Melanie was going to have her incision, then bandaged the same spot, to show her how she'd look afterward. They'd talked about her going to sleep while the doctor made the bad bump go away. Melanie used her new doll for demonstration purposes, and I didn't miss the irony of her explaining all of this to me in her self-assured, four-year-old voice.

Will kissed us goodbye and left for work. He'd come back by to have supper with me, then I'd take the car home to be with the baby while he stayed the night. Melanie and I snuggled on her bed and read books and sang songs. When the anesthesiologist came by and talked to her about getting a needle to go to sleep for a while the next morning, she was unconcerned. She'd gone to sleep like that once before, when she had her tonsils out. Would she get popsicles this time too?

I think her confidence kept me calm. Margaret and I had agreed not to call just to check in, so the fact that the phone didn't ring was a plus. My breasts were tight and sore to the touch; I'd nursed Gregg right before I left that morning, but he usually ate about four times before three in the afternoon. I had to change the soggy pads in my bra often, reminding me each time that I couldn't feed my baby, but I was dealing with that. My focus was on my daughter. When I went out in the hall for a break, other mothers were there with their children, some in wheelchairs, one little girl in a shopping cart. A nurse's aide told me that child had spina bifida. I tried to focus on how lucky we'd been, having exactly the right pediatrician who knew exactly the right medical expert who knew exactly the right surgeon to operate on Melanie, but it's hard to see the upside of your four-year-old daughter going into a surgery that could leave one side of her face paralyzed.

That night I drove home after Will got to the hospital to stay with Melanie. I must've been on autopilot. Margaret, uncomplaining, was clearly exhausted, and Gregg was beside himself. His face was wet, his nose was running, his skinny arms were flailing as his grandmother held him. I took him up to our room. Without the need to talk, we all went to bed. Margaret needed her sleep, and Gregg needed to nurse. I slept little that night, between his feedings and my fears. I made more breastmilk bottles, and before the sun was up, I fed him and woke Margaret so I could leave for the hospital.

The morning was dim and foggy. Though leaves were falling, autumn had not really begun. Days were still mild, nights muggy. Driving into the city, across the old 14th Street Bridge, no other cars around, was eerie, otherworldly. When I got to the room, Will was asleep in a chair, and Melanie wasn't awake yet. I envied their calm. In only minutes the medical machine cranked up, though, and before I was ready, we were wheeling her into the operating arena. We were able to stay while she counted backward, so she'd see us as she fell asleep. Then the waiting began.

In a little over two hours, a nurse came out to tell us Melanie was doing fine. After two more hours, the surgeon came out smiling, and the breath I'd been holding for weeks, it seemed, let go. We stood, but he made us sit as he told us the surgery had been a total success. The nerve ganglion was touch and go, but he'd extracted the diseased lymph node without causing any permanent nerve damage.

"Don't be alarmed at the way her face droops for the next few weeks or so. She's going to heal up nicely; you'll never notice her scar, unless you look for it."

When she woke, the whole left side of her face looked like she had palsy; it drooped like the unstitched hem of a skirt. But she rallied with little pain or nausea, and her stay in the hospital to recuperate was pretty uneventful—except for my nightly treks back and forth to feed the baby and try to get a little sleep.

One day I'll never forget: Melanie was up and around, eating well, and wanted to go to the playroom. Her nurses gave the okay, so I went with her, concerned she might be weaker than she realized. When we got there, a little boy about her age was sitting in front of the TV screen, his back to us. Melanie, in one of her feminine nightgowns, delighted to have another child to talk to after all the adults, tapped him on the shoulder, said, "Whatcha watchin?" When he turned, most of his face looked as if it had been melted away. He was a recovering burn victim, in for another round of skin grafts. We were so lucky.

Despite Melanie's surgery and Gregg's uneasy transition into our family, we surely had the worst behind us, I figured. We could move forward pretty unscathed, unlike that little boy who'd always wear his scars. When we took Melanie home the next day, and Margaret, more exhausted than she'd admit, left, I welcomed a return to normalcy. We'd survived some bad times, but they both could've been far worse; the troubles were behind us now and we were all okay. Even if Will and I didn't communicate so well, we'd gotten through these tough things together somehow. Enough already; it was past time for the four of us to settle in as a typical, uncomplicated family.

CHAPTER 3 -- THE BAD WOMAN

We moved twice in the next year and a half. Paying rent and keeping the baby in a converted closet weren't ideal. Carmen and her family bought a house in Sugarland, on the outskirts of Reston, Virginia. We liked that less congested area of the D.C. metropolis a lot. Plus Carmen was my only gal pal close by. We put a down payment on a condo in Herndon, the next planned community over from them, in the first section of the development. We moved when Gregg was six months old.

That first fall Melanie started country-day school with her buddy Christy, Carmen's older girl. The little yellow school bus picked her up and dropped her off at our front door. Gregg was an easy-going baby. He'd caught up physically, and though he was behind Melanie's developmental markers, the doctors assured us he was well within normal range for a boy. The friendly couple next door had a baby, too, and I enjoyed coffee every now and then with the mom. We intended to stay in Herndon a while, to settle in. A couple of events changed our minds.

A white policeman shot a Black man at the 7-Eleven just beyond the entrance to our neighborhood. The unrest turned to violence, and the old mansion intended for renovation as our community center mysteriously burned one night.

A neighbor, a German woman who'd been an Army bride, offered, "If you want, I have an extra pistol," since Will was gone so much, usually twelve hours a day. His drive each way to his office was over an hour. As a civil engineer, he was a project manager, and that took him on lots of job sites even farther away.

I blanched at the thought of a weapon in the house and murmured a feeble, "Ah, no thanks. I'll see what Will wants to do." As tensions subsided, I worried less, but my image of an idyllic semi-rural lifestyle had been shattered.

The construction company Will worked for was a partnership, owned by two older engineers. He had a great salary, terrific benefits, and lots of autonomy on his jobs. Unexpectedly that spring, Will came home early.

"Mr. Whitehead died. Of a heart attack."

"What's Mr. Leech gonna do? He'll keep the company going, won't he?"

"We'll have to wait and see," he said.

We were shocked to find out the company was in financial disarray. Will decided the safest thing to do was look for a new job, just in case. Within weeks, he found a terrific opportunity working with a young high-powered company in Richmond. He took the offer and bought a house in my old neighborhood, contingent on my approval, and before I knew it we were on our way back "home."

Before we left, Carmen and I went out to lunch without the children, a sort of girl's goodbye fling. Though we never drank during the day, we had a few beers with our meal. We noticed that a couple of attractive men nearby were flirting with us, and we giggled like college girls at the attention.

One came over and offered to buy us drinks—"Hello, ladies—how ya handling that big thirst? Could I buy you a round?" We laughed so hard we probably scared him off before we could get out our no thanks. Later, I wondered why I'd felt so flattered, rather than offended, by strange males being attracted to me. Why did that feel good? But I didn't give it much thought, just enjoyed the sexy little secret.

Moving twice was a strain, but I was over the moon to be out of D.C. It didn't hold many happy memories for me. Our new pediatrician, Dr. Kendig, had interned under my own childhood physician, Dr. Anderson, who used to come to the house when my brothers or I had a fever. I had complete confidence in him.

My grandmother and aunt lived in Richmond; my parents were only a few blocks away. One brother was in the Air Force in Spain, another was working in Panama, but I had plenty of childhood friendships to renew, and Will and I had a couple of friends from college, too. This move felt right in every way. Finally, we could get our family—and our relationship—on track.

Gregg was a year old, still not walking or talking, but a lovable chunk of a child. He smiled all the time, and by this time, he was happy to go to his dad for his bottle. He laughed when we tickled him and kicked our arms away when we changed his diapers. He crawled all over the place and sat up to build blocks and play Fisher-Price toolbox.

But he didn't ever babble or cry much, and he still didn't sleep all night. Our friend Andy called him "blivet," some description in his mind that suited Gregg to a T. I called him my Sugar Crisp Sugar Bear. One of his favorite toys was his set of Weebles; we'd laugh and say, "Weebles wobble but they don't fall down." Gregg reminded me of those Weebles in more ways than one.

More than four years apart, Melanie and Gregg were rarely together, except at mealtime. She was a jabberer, he content to sit in his high-chair and eat his food or play with his spoon. I was pleased she'd never behaved as if she were jealous of him. On the other hand, she'd never paid much attention to him either. In the fall, she started kindergarten a few blocks from our new home.

Will could drop her off on the way to work, and Gregg and I had our quiet days at home.

One major problem persevered: Gregg woke up at least once a night, usually twice. We tried a mini-meal right before bed, like oatmeal and bananas. He'd have a bath, and I'd read and sing to him and give him his "last" bottle and food. He relaxed right down to sleep, but then woke up around two or three, restless and wanting more milk. He'd drink all eight ounces down, so I didn't think I could deny it. Dr. Kendig recommended medication, even paregoric, but I was unwilling to "drug" him. Will was working, I wasn't, so it seemed only fair that I was the one to get up and give him a nighttime bottle. Sleep deprivation sapped my energy, until most days I was on emotional autopilot, but I worked hard to put a happy face on my situation. Gregg didn't sleep through the night for the first seventeen months of his life. I should have given him medication; in hindsight, I should have been in therapy myself, certainly, but I never gave it a thought. All my energy went to getting through the days and nights taking care of my two children.

Gregg still had health problems, too. He had a terrible bronchial sounding cough. The doctor called it bronchial asthma. When it got bad at night, Gregg would lose his breath, and we'd have to take him into the bathroom, turn on the shower as hot as it would go, and hold him and pat his back while the steam opened up his breathing passages. This rudimentary solution to my child not being able to breathe made me feel helpless and terrified, but it worked.

One night at supper, sitting in his high-chair in the kitchen, Gregg pushed back so hard he knocked the chair over. His head hit the radiator under the window, and it split. Will and I jumped into the car, me holding a towel to Gregg's head to staunch the bleeding (we must've taken Melanie to a neighbor's), and raced to the emergency room. They rushed him into an examination room right away; he required stitches. The doctor said he showed no signs of a concussion, so we took him home, grateful the damage was minor. I don't remember them taking x-rays, but they did.

My anxiety and irritability mounted, and I directed my dissatisfaction at my marriage. I spent a lot of time on church activities, trying to get some spiritual grounding. At first, to try to soften the tension, I flailed around for some hobby away from home that would be all mine and had nothing to do with Will or the children. For some reason, I landed on horseback riding, never thinking for a second how stereotypical adolescent girl that was. My close friend Nancy told me of a stable in Hanover near her farm, and one day I drove out there to meet the riding instructor. He was a courtly older man with a British accent and intelligent blue eyes. He looked like my mental image of a horse person, and I liked his ease with himself and the animals and his openness with me. After touring the stables, he told me the fees, scheduled my first lesson, and gave me a list of the gear I would need and where to buy it. The boots alone cost $85, but I loved how tall and slender I looked in the tan riding pants and black boots up to the knee.

And the lessons excited me. The instructor said I was a natural; I learned to post and trot right away. Being up on an enormous horse was scary and powerful at the same time. After a couple of lessons, I felt certain I'd made the right choice. But my instructor's hands began to linger a bit longer than seemed necessary on my butt when he was helping me with posture. I ignored this, blaming my hypersensitivity. I wasn't a big fan of cantering or galloping, but I breezed along and he kept advancing my skill levels. When he introduced jumping, I told him I didn't want to do that. I only wanted to ride. He claimed I'd love it once I got the feel, and that it was an essential aspect of English riding. At his insistence, I took a couple of jumps, scared senseless though they were barely off the ground. That last lesson he made way more eye contact than before.

When it was over, he walked the horse back to its stall with me and suggested, "Might you like to come out for an evening ride? The trails are amazing at sunset." Even in my clueless bubble, I had to admit to myself that he was coming on to me. I have no way of knowing for certain, but I didn't go back. That male attention rattled me in a wonky approach-avoidance way that I didn't want to examine too closely.

I did go back to work part-time, certain I'd be a better wife if I weren't homebound. My mother and Will's mom had both worked; this was not a conflict for us. One of my high school buddies, George, had married the brightest, most positive young woman, Carol J. They had two children, a boy and a girl a bit older than Gregg, and the boy was in school. Carol wanted to stay home—she loved being a stay-at-home mom—but she wanted to make some money, too. And she adored Gregg. He went to her easily, which put my mind at ease. So Gregg spent my work hours with Carol and her four-year-old daughter, and I went back to teaching, beginning with tutoring reading a few hours a day.

Gregg loved it there. Carol was such a sparkly mom-person. She was the creative type who planned age-appropriate activities every day. Her perky pleasure with the children was a clear contrast to my crankiness. This was right for us, for me, for our family. Around thirteen months, Gregg started walking; at fifteen months, he began to talk—"juice, cookie" were his first words—and shortly after he finally started to sleep each night. From thereon, though, he never did take afternoon naps, but that was a small price for me to pay for a full night's rest. I was much happier. We all were.

After a semester part-time, my friend Julia Ann, who was working at a secondary school for adolescents with dyslexia, suggested I apply for a position teaching language there. I jumped at the chance. I'd been an English major in college, and though I taught first grade for five years, I'd always wanted to work with older children.

My job was more like college than work. The teachers were from all over—New York, Massachusetts, Connecticut, Jamaica.

The training was intensive. I spent nights studying, days teaching, and considerable after-school time asking the other teachers questions. This new circle of colleagues fast became friends. I was developing a fulfilling life apart from Will. At home, the children got my left-over energy; little was expended on my husband or my marriage. Will was busy, too, with project plans spread out on the dining room table evenings, intent on sealing his position with his new company. We never bickered, never argued; we were considerate of one another, committed to our children, and well-matched as sexual partners. But somewhere back when Gregg was born we'd lost that elusive connection we'd had early on.

I didn't worry about it, though. I felt more mentally alive than I had in years, what with brain theory and instructional experimentation and conversation with well-traveled colleagues. Maybe this was the way marriages worked, more like loving friends. I decided I was happiest when I had things to think about outside the family, so I signed up to take summer courses. There was so much for me to learn about this new field, teaching English and reading to teens with dyslexia. Carol was happy to have Gregg all year-round, and I was happy to be Charlotte the Professional.

Two things happened to jar our somewhat serene, though unstimulating, lives: Carol and George moved, and my friend Nancy developed breast cancer again.

Before they moved an hour away, Carol helped me figure out a situation for Gregg that we thought might work. Another gal in the neighborhood, Betty, had a son Gregg's age, Kevin. They'd played together some. Kevin was boisterous and his mom's parenting style was more laid-back than either mine or Carol's, but I liked her well enough and thought it might be helpful for Gregg to have a more outgoing boy to interact with. We decided we would give it a try.

The new situation was a disaster. Gregg came home unhappy. He complained Kevin was rough. When I talked to Betty, she said they were only playing. But Gregg didn't want to go there in the morning. This had never happened before when we were going to Carol's. Now he'd dawdle and say he didn't like it at Betty's. Her house was in disarray, with toys everywhere and old paint cans and ladders all over the place from half-finished home renovation projects, and papers and books and dishes covering every surface. Carol and I were both no-clutter freaks. Plus it just seemed grey every time I walked into that living room, though the house was full of windows. The vibes weren't right. The last day he stayed there, Gregg was sitting on the sofa crying quiet tears when I came to pick him up after school. Kevin was galloping around the coffee table.

"What's wrong, Boog?" I asked. He shrugged his little shoulders. "Betty?"

"I don't know," she apologized. "He was like this all day."

"Why didn't you call me?"

"He didn't have a fever or anything." It was her turn to shrug. "He wouldn't eat his lunch, either."

I picked Gregg up, saddled him onto my hip. "This isn't going to work."

"Okay." Her blasé attitude infuriated me.

Gregg held onto me and we got out of there. I was mad enough to spit: at Betty, at myself, at my situation. I needed to work, but what could I do with him? He was one of those children who had a hard time shifting gears, adapting.

Daycare was my problem since Will would've been just as happy for me to stay home. I had to find a positive situation for Gregg, and find it fast. I'd never thought about putting him in a daycare facility. I liked having him close to home in a homey situation, with only a child or two beside him, given his quiet nature and lack of assertiveness. But another friend, Carol S., described this school out in the country where her two children had gone, and she was a no-nonsense mom who would have never tolerated inappropriate or slack behavior from the childcare provider. I needed help fast, I respected Carol S. as a friend and a mother, and I didn't have any more satisfactory alternative at hand, so I drove out there to take a look. The place was cheerful, inviting, and clean. The teachers and aides were pleasant and approachable. The playground was safe, with plenty of different equipment for the different age groups. I talked to the director about Gregg, about nutrition, about hours and costs. This would be it, then. I would bring Gregg starting the next week.

Neither of us liked the added rush in the morning or the twenty-five-minute drive out. Gregg was a child who couldn't be rushed. He would be agreeable—"I'm getting dressed now, Mom"—but he did everything at Gregg-speed. So the daycare change upped the tension level at home. I had to be at work by eight, so we needed to leave the house by 7:15 at the latest. Will had started leaving even earlier for job sites—around 6:30, usually—so I was dropping Melanie off, too, and she didn't like going that early.

"I don't see why Gregg has to go out to the country every day." It was not a good start to the day for the three of us.

When Nancy's cancer recurred that spring, the oncologist recommended surgery immediately. Right before she'd gone on a trip to Hawaii, I'd been with her while she tried on bathing suits. On the side where she'd had the mastectomy, just above her reconstructed breast, she'd felt a lump. She had me check, and I could feel it, too. Her skin was a bit discolored, bruised looking.

"You'd better see about that," I'd advised.

"I will, when I get back from my trip," she'd answered. "Besides, there's no breast tissue left, so I couldn't have breast cancer." We'd even laughed.

After this most recent surgery, she needed more treatments. They put her in the hospital for weeks at a time, and she hated to be there at night alone. I volunteered with a couple of other close friends to come spend the night with her a couple of nights a week.

"You think you ought to do that?" Will asked. He loved Nancy almost as much as I did, and he respected our friendship, but he was worried. "You're already stretched to the max, with school and the kids. Andy can afford a night nurse." His concern was genuine, I'm sure, but I'm stubborn. My best friend needed her best friend. I wasn't about to say no.

"It's not the same. She wants a friend there. I'll be fine. I'll come home early enough in the morning to shower and get ready for school. You're gonna have to do night duty, though."

He agreed to two nights a week, and I began my shifts staying with her.

Will was right, though. I was on overload. I blocked out the fact that I wasn't spending enough time with my children. While I'm sure my subconscious guilt factory was active, I told myself this was the right thing to do. Will was a grown man; he was their daddy. At this stage in their lives, he could do anything I could do. But mornings after I'd been with Nancy, Gregg would cling to me.

"Can we stay home today, Mama?" I'd take homework to the hospital, and after Nancy went to sleep I'd do my school papers. I was spread too thin, but wouldn't admit it.

One morning when I came home around 6:30, needing to take a shower and get ready for school, Will met me at the door. "This isn't working. You need to be home with us." My throat tightened, like I was going to cry.

"That's not fair," I yelled. I was never one to raise my voice, but I did.

"Shhh," he warned. "The kids are still upstairs. They don't need to hear you."

I hated disapproval and couldn't deal with personal criticism. I didn't want to cry, either, to look like I was at my wit's end, which I was.

"You are so right," I forced out. "This is NOT working." I started up the stairs.

"Charlotte, we need to talk," he said, but I wouldn't turn around. I cried in the shower, and then I got myself and Gregg ready for school.

"What's wrong, Mama?" he wanted to know.

"I'm fine, Boog, just really really tired. Okay?"

"Okay."

I wasn't scheduled to go back to the hospital to spend the night for four or five days, so the flare-up died down and we didn't talk about it. Nancy got better, she went home, and we settled into our family roles again that summer and fall. Will and I occasionally got a babysitter and did a couple things, but not much. Mostly we had family cookouts or get-togethers with our friends who had children close in age to ours. On the surface, we were any happily married couple with children, but I wasn't satisfied at all. I wanted something more, something different, but I didn't even know what that might be.

One day, when my mother and stepfather were over for a meal, I took my mother upstairs under the pretense of showing her something one of the children had made. She'd divorced my daddy when I was about eight and my younger brother was six. Surely she'd understand my dilemma and could give me good advice.

I sat her down on my bed and said, "I'm thinking about getting a divorce."

"What?" she almost yelled.

I patted her knee. "Nothing's wrong, Mama, it's just that..."

"Well if nothing's wrong, why would you even think such a thing?"

I pressed on. "Will's not having an affair or anything. Neither am I. But we're not compatible . . ."

"Don't be silly, Charlotte." She smiled, but her voice had an edge. "Why in the world would you even say such a thing?"

"That's not what I mean. I'm not happy, and I feel lonesome a lot."

"Will is a good man, and he's great with Melanie and Gregg. What would you do without him?"

"I don't know. I could—"

"All I can say is you'd better think long and hard about it. It's not easy being a single mother. I should know. Your daddy never sent me a penny."

"But Mama, I'm so sad all the time."

"Well get a hobby. When I'm sad I go work in the garden. Your yard could use some attention."

"Maybe I don't love him."

"You loved him when you got married, didn't you? You were the one who just had to get married your last year of college."

"You know he had to go in the Army, and we were scared he'd get sent to Vietnam . . ."

"That's beside the point. If you loved him once, you'll love him again. Just set your mind on it. Those children need a daddy, take my word." She stood up.

"Oh Mama, I don't know what to do."

She gave me a hug, held me back so she could look me in the eye. "Give it some time. Promise me you'll give it some time. You're a smart girl, Charlotte. Don't do anything you'll regret. You've always rushed into things."

"Okay. I guess you're right." I didn't know what else to say. We went back downstairs to join the men and children.

One day soon after that conversation, Will showed me a copy of a review in *Time* magazine of Maribel Morgan's *Total Woman*, a "how-to" book for married women advocating not only deference to the husband, but also claiming that the woman in the marriage was responsible for everything from eggs to beds.

He said, smiling, "Maybe you ought to read that book." I knew he was teasing, and he didn't really want me to wrap myself in Saran Wrap and meet him naked at the front door, but I couldn't go along with his joke. I socked it away as just another sign that he didn't understand me a single teensy bit, rather than an effort on his part to be lighthearted.

That winter I flirted outrageously with our minister. I was the chair of Christian Education at our church, and our young priest was handsome, smart, lively, and innovative. Talking with him about movies and books and ethical issues was like all these electric switches lit up all over my body and brain. I adored his wife, too, but against my will, I developed a crush on him. I went to see him for marriage counseling, and sparks flew. He told me he found me seductive, too, and he'd been thinking about me recently in "that way." We met a number of times in his office to talk about our marriages and why we might be sexually attracted to one another, and even took a walk one day on the wooded church grounds and kissed in that way that demanded more. To my dismay, he set up a meeting between me and Will and his wife, so the four of us could take a look together at the problems in each marriage that might be causing the two of us to "lust in our hearts."

Will went to the session; he was understanding and forgiving. He'd do anything to make the marriage work. The priest's wife was as calm as a Buddha. It was all civilized and unemotional and unsatisfying. I was mortified. Will and I started counseling with a religious-based therapist, and we were no more than three weeks into our session before the man sent Will home and told me I was depressed and we wouldn't get anywhere until he dealt with me in one-on-one sessions.

Me, depressed? Certainly not. I was unhappy in my marriage, yes, stretched too thin with two children and a full-time job teaching teenagers, okay, but what made him think I was depressed? I was not ready to hear what he had to say. I'd come to counseling to work on my marriage, which I was not at all certain we could save.

The guy tried to reach me, I give him credit for that, but we weren't a good match. I stopped going. Will and I lived with the status quo: going about our lives as a married couple, without talking about my fears and anxieties and loneliness. Without talking much at all, really.

The children were both great. I was good at putting on a smiling demeanor, and they did make me happy. Melanie's teachers were certain she'd grow up to be the first female president. After school, she'd go to my neighbors two doors down to play with her best friend Kara, her exact age. Gregg had a little trouble adjusting to his new daycare situation. The teachers wanted him to take a nap, like all the four-year-olds, but he wouldn't. He hadn't taken naps for two years, I told them. We reached a compromise: they pulled his cot into a storage room during rest period, where he could look at books or color as long as he was quiet. I didn't like him being isolated like that, but they weren't willing to let him stay if he disrupted naptime. This wasn't ideal, but his whole not napping was going to be a problem anywhere, even at home, so we made do.

That winter I took longer and longer picking him up. I'd stay after school to work until the very last minute, or go out for a beer at a neighborhood bar with some of my fellow teachers. Many of them were single; most had traveled or been to school outside Virginia, and talking to them gave me a sense that my life had been so small. We laughed and discussed politics and education and relationships, and when I was with them, I felt like I was connected, that I had a brain. At home, I played with my children and cooked suppers and did laundry, feeling dead inside.

I made it through Christmas, but in January, I felt like I couldn't breathe, so I asked Will to move out. He was floored, but I wouldn't change my mind or go back to therapy. I'd been unhappy too long. I'd tried the ridiculous to the sublime: horseback riding, flirting, going back to school, getting a job. For me, somehow, everything pointed to the fact that my marriage wasn't an emotional cushion, a place where I could talk through my thoughts and be understood, be comforted, and offer comfort, my safe haven with my life partner. We didn't fit, no matter how hard we tried. Maybe I hadn't been fair, maybe I hadn't talked to him about it enough, but I didn't see how it could ever change if we stayed together.

He sought someone's help himself. He was kind to me, trying to get me to talk, scheduling childcare so we could go out to a movie and dinner, things I liked to do. One night in a restaurant, after we'd been to see *The Deep*, I was paralyzed over my meal. I literally couldn't put a bite of food in my mouth. I felt like I was about to choke.

He took my hand, tried to be tender and understanding— "Come on, Charlotte. We'll be fine. I promise."—but it was over for me, and I couldn't bear dragging it out. I weighed less than a hundred pounds, I wasn't sleeping, the effort to be a good mom to my children was getting harder and harder, and I never wanted to reach a point where I ignored them or their needs. He agreed to find an apartment and move out, but he assured me he wasn't giving up on us.

That Saturday we sat the children down in the living room to tell them we were separating, that Daddy was moving out. "Your daddy loves you; he'll always be your daddy. You'll spend lots of fun time with him still. The only thing that'll be different is that he'll live in a different place. You can go over there some times, once he gets settled." Will, Melanie, and Gregg were crying. I was the only one who could talk. "We both promise you, you're going to be fine. You're still going to have a mama and a daddy who love you."

"When?" Melanie wanted to know.

"Soon. Real soon," I answered, and all three of them cried even more. What was wrong with me? How could I sit here and talk about the break-up of my family and feel so empty inside? With this man who had been nothing but understanding? I knew I had to do this, that I'd destroy myself in some awful way if I didn't, but I still couldn't make it right. That old saying of my grandmother's—it's bound to get worse before it gets better—was my only consolation.

Will found a small apartment not too far away, and he started having the children sleep over on weekends. He did well with them, taking them to ballgames and for pizza or Mexican food or out to Nancy and Andy's farm. But when he'd come back Sunday evenings, he'd want to stay, and they'd want him to stay, and I had to be the one to say no all over again. Common wisdom says it takes two to make a marriage and two to break one, too, but I knew that this failure belonged to me. I didn't miss him, didn't miss our life together, but I still wasn't happy. My guilt was all over the place. My mother told me I was making a big mistake. Will's brother and sister-in-law, the nicest two people on Earth, called from Arkansas to tell me how sorry they were that we were separated, how they understood I'd been having a rough time, and to please know I could call to talk to them any time. Everyone was so good except me—I was the bad woman who'd wrecked her marriage and family for no tangible reason. I couldn't even deal with it myself.

On weekends when the children were with Will, I began going out with my school friends. We'd get together in a big group, couples and singles, at someone's house or a bar to listen to music or dance or just talk. One man in particular, the artist-in-residence, would sit with me and talk about movies and art and children. He had a son himself, but he'd been divorced for almost six years. I enjoyed getting to know him, but I was in no way on the lookout for a romance.

The semester rolled along like that. Will gave me two concert tickets to see Kris Kristofferson, but I took Carol S. He invited me out to dinner for my birthday, and I went, thinking we needed to be able to spend time together, for Gregg and Melanie, but when he took me home I couldn't let him stay. It wouldn't have been right. He did everything conceivable to heal our broken family, but I was incapable of renewing my marriage with him. I knew in my heart that I couldn't live that way, that it was over between us. I couldn't make it right.

Gregg's daycare graduation occurred one bright summer afternoon. Parents were invited to see the little ones get their "diplomas" and have cookies and juice afterward. We were outside, the sun was shining but not too hot, and I had a sense that things would work out, eventually, even though I had no idea how.

After the brief ceremony, I was standing by myself while Gregg horsed around with some of his friends. He didn't hang on me much anymore, which pleased me. One of the aides, a woman I'd seen often but hadn't officially met, walked up to me. "Are you Gregg's mother?" she asked.

"Why yes, I am," I answered, smiling.

"Could I talk to you for just a moment? About Gregg?"

"Sure." We stepped away from the noisy children.

"I feel like I have to say this. I hope you won't be upset. But I need to tell you: Gregg's an angry little boy."

"What?" I lost my breath.

"I just thought you ought to know."

She walked away, leaving me with the sensation that I'd had the wind knocked out of me. Gregg NEVER threw tantrums, never hit other children or took their toys, never complained. A sweet-natured child, he hardly cried, unless he was physically hurt. Usually, there had to be blood for him to so much as whimper. He was dear to me, patting my cheek, kissing me good night, telling me he loved me. I didn't know what to make of what this woman said. Except it hit a raw nerve.

I went up and hugged him goodbye—he was going with his dad for the weekend—and he had a big smile on his face, his cheeks all pink from playing. He looked like the most normal, healthy, happy boy in the world. But when I got in my car I cried and cried, all that crying I hadn't let go for the past four years.

CHAPTER 4 -- OUR EASY CHILD

I married the next spring, to the artist-colleague at my school. Many people, Will included, thought we'd been having an affair all along, and he could blame our divorce on that, but we hadn't. We'd been friends, close friends, until one spring day we realized we were in love. The day of our reception, at our new home together, Gregg and his new stepbrother Jaison, two years older, supposedly brawled on the front lawn. Melanie, a little brainiac in glasses, told everyone who would listen that she hated her new stepfather. But I was in love and for once happy with myself and my life choices, and I considered these childish behaviors predictable and no cause for concern. John was as fair and devoted with my two children as he was with his own son, who lived with us in our custody.

The five of us moved into his home in Ashland; John and I knew we had to expect blended-family problems, but we talked all the time about everything from art history to yard sales, and we had total confidence that working as loving equals, we could make our lives together work. I'd regained my self-confidence and optimism; I was over the hump.

Gregg was our easy child. Melanie could be sharp-tongued, lording her intelligence over the two boys, who were both equally smart but less verbal and assertive.

She'd tease Jaison, who was a beautiful boy. "Your haircut looks like a girl's." She'd call Gregg a brat and accuse him of being a dummy. Jaison, a happy-go-lucky clown of a boy, would get in minor trouble in school. One day he'd actually skipped first grade. Regimen didn't suit him, and teachers would call to complain about him drawing when he was supposed to be doing math, or whispering and making faces during silent reading. The two older ones were often assigned punishments, but Gregg rarely got in trouble.

Of course he had flare-ups. The first Easter we were together, John dyed a blown egg for Melanie. It was all swirled pastels, one of a kind. She put it with her treasures, in with her doll collection. He gave the boys something else—a chocolate bunny and baseball cards for each, nothing he'd made. A few days later I heard Melanie and Gregg arguing in her room. She came through the kitchen and went out back to play Barbies. I was relieved that they'd settled whatever they were bickering about by themselves. Later, when she went back to her room, she screamed for me.

"Mama. Come here now! Come see what Gregg did!" He'd smashed her egg. I sat him down and talked to him and made him apologize to her, then gave him time out, but she was furious with him for destroying her beautiful, unique gift.

That fall we decided to have Gregg repeat kindergarten. He had a late birthday, and he hadn't liked school at all that first year. Sometimes he would hide under the table when the reading teacher came for him. He was ahead of the other children academically, but he was short and socially immature.

One day when I'd been driving him to school he'd asked, "Mama, instead of going to school to teach, why can't you stay home and teach me?" I hated that, but now I had to work. As a full-time practicing artist, John only worked as a teacher part-time, so his regular salary was not enough for the five of us to live on. My child-support was minuscule, but my lawyer had advised against challenging it. Will had agreed to pay for college for both children, and that benefit alone was worth a lot. But monthly economics were tight, and I couldn't stop working full-time.

Gregg hated being held back. It played into his sense of being "dumber" than his lively, bright, verbal siblings. But he was the athlete of the family. Short, he had the build of a bull-calf. He could throw a Frisbee, hit a baseball, run as fast as the older two. In Little League his first year, he had an unassisted triple play, when he was six years old. That made the Richmond sports page. That same year, he scored five unassisted goals in one game playing soccer. He always got praise for his sports prowess. I was satisfied that each of the children had an individual way to shine: Melanie was the intellectual, Jaison had the winning personality, and Gregg was the super athlete.

He viewed the world in unexpected ways, too. Once, he called John into the bathroom. "Johnnnn (he'd draw his words out, as though he were meditating at the same time he was talking), does poop turn to mud?" Another time, riding in the back seat while John and I were in front, he asked, out of the blue, "Why does George Washington have that ball on the back of his head?" Another time, when he was taking Benadryl for his stuffy nose, he woke up in the night and called for me. John went in to him. "Guess what, John? I floated up to the ceiling."

"You did? What did you do then?"

"I just floated back down." He was an oddball original thinker. I saw this as a plus, and in first grade, when the school did the initial standardized testing for his class, Gregg's scores put him in the "genius" category. Johns Hopkins notified us that he was eligible for their early-identification-program for math gifted children. Unfortunately, we didn't have the extra money to take advantage of their programs.

For all his athletic prowess, Gregg couldn't swim or float, and this caused him grief in our water-loving family. Our home was on the Randolph-Macon College campus, and the children had use of the gym and swimming pool when classes or athletics weren't scheduled. He and Jaison would go over and shoot baskets, and Gregg was a dead-eye. Melanie wouldn't go, mostly because she didn't do anything she didn't do well. She swam like a dolphin, though, with grace, speed, and natural agility. Jaison swam like a competitor, no pretty strokes, but he could cut through the water. But because of his muscular build, Gregg was a cinderblock in the pool. John had been a water safety instructor, so he committed himself to teaching Gregg to swim. The others laughed at him as he flailed in the pool, not moving forward an inch. When he'd lie on his back to float, inevitably he ended up vertical instead of horizontal. He had no fear and wouldn't give up; he'd put his head down and move his arms and legs, making every physical effort to swim, but he'd sink. Tenacious, he'd go over day after day and get water-logged trying, but he couldn't get the hang of it.

One day John said, "Listen, Gregg, if you can swim the width of the pool, I'll take you to K & K Toys and you can pick out any toy in the entire store." Jaison and Melanie actually cheered him on, and Gregg did it. He learned to swim that day. True to his promise, John drove the three of them into Richmond to go to the shopping center. That night he told me, "I thought I'd jump out of my skin waiting for Gregg to decide what he wanted. He walked up and down every aisle, looked at everything, wouldn't let any of us tell him what to get. He took over an hour to make up his mind, and you know what he got? One of those little Star Wars figures that cost a dollar ninety-eight." Melanie and Jaison teased him all the way home for being "such a dolt." Nobody could make up Gregg's mind for him; he had his own unique, quiet, curious way of being in the world. He had never been a follower.

To say he was a quiet child would be an understatement, but in our boisterous family, I was grateful for one listener. His silence created consequences, though. The first day he went to school in Ashland, he took the school bus. When the kids got off the bus at the end of the day, he didn't get off with Jaison. John called me at work in Richmond to say he'd called the school, but they had no idea where he was. I panicked, but he told me not to worry; he'd call the school board office and figure out what was going on. Sure enough, he called back about fifteen minutes later. Gregg was in the office at the local high school. The bus driver had finished her elementary school run and had gone to the high school for her second run. When she stood up to take a break, there was this little boy, Gregg, sitting near the back. He hadn't made a peep. He had no idea where he was. At supper that night, Melanie and Jaison thought this was a riot. Gregg didn't find it so funny.

He did get the best of them once. In the woods behind our house, they'd apparently jerry-rigged a fort of sorts, dragging some kind of chest back there where they stored supplies, including *Playboys* and other girlie magazines. They'd filched these from trashcans at the college dorms bordering our property behind our backyard. We knew nothing of the fort or the magazines.

One night at the table Gregg, almost six, piped up, "I wanna know something." We all listened. "I can understand why guys like to look at naked girls up here"—he pointed to his chest; Melanie and Jaison started yelling, "Gregg!" and "Shut up!" John and I shushed them. He continued, "but why do they want to look at them down here." He pointed to his crotch. John and I had to stifle laughs. We tried to explain that grown people did a lot of things that were private that might be confusing to children. And what made him think that people looked at those things anyway? The whole fort story came out. We made them tear it down, confiscated the magazines, and destroyed them, and Melanie and Jaison were furious with Gregg for weeks.

In first grade his teacher didn't like him for some reason I never understood. She was a sharp, attractive young woman who ran a pretty tight classroom, and Gregg didn't fit into her picture of what a six-year-old boy should be. He could do the math problems too fast, he didn't like reading books, he didn't always answer questions right away, he was slow to follow instructions. These didn't strike me as serious offenses, but somehow they added up to an awkward relationship between those two.

One fall day, the school called me at work in Richmond. It was the office, reporting the teacher's concern (outrage?) because the day was chilly, and Gregg had come to school in shirtsleeves. Was I aware of this? She was worried about letting him go out for recess without a jacket. He begged to play outside. Of course I was aware of it. I was his mother. Gregg had hated being swaddled as an infant and would squirm out of a blanket every time we covered him. He couldn't stand big bulky coats and never wore anything too heavy, even on the coldest day. I wouldn't press him about his temperature gauge. I told the secretary to send back word that he had my permission to go out with the group. If he needed a coat he'd wear a coat. I'm afraid I didn't earn too many points with that teacher, either.

At the end of the year, she had a policy of taking the child with the highest average (average what, in first grade?) out to lunch as a reward for work well done. Gregg won, and they went out for pizza together; he got to choose the place.

The children's lives continued to change. Will remarried a year after I did, to Betti, a special ed teacher with a sweet-natured son only a year younger than Gregg. As they settled in as a family, I was hopeful that Gregg and his new stepbrother would become good friends, and he would grow close to his dad as well. This didn't happen. In fact, though he thought his stepbrother was friendly and lots of fun, and those two always enjoyed being together, Gregg grew to dislike his new stepmother, and from a distance, it appeared the feeling was mutual. Melanie, ever anxious to please her daddy, knew when to put on the charm and when she could get away with being stubborn or ill-tempered. And Will was justifiably proud of her, so she and Betti made an uneasy truce. Gregg never learned much social maneuvering, that just wasn't his nature, and he couldn't do anything to please the "step monster," as they both called her. On Sunday nights when he'd get home from a weekend at his dad's, he'd talk to me about the way she treated him. When Betti asked him to help bring in the groceries, he was too slow; she labeled this as "laziness." When his dad brought him a gift, say a new baseball glove, he didn't ooh and ahh; she noted this as "ingratitude." At the dinner table when he didn't join in the talk, she called this "sullen," or even worse, "rude." To his young eyes, his dad would do whatever Betti said; he would always take her side against him. This made Gregg sad, and some nights when he got home from his dad's, he cried about it when he was alone in bed.

"I wish my daddy still liked me." This, the guy who never cried when he hurt.

When Will and I talked on the phone about the children, our conversations became tense. He didn't think I was strict enough with Melanie and Gregg. To my mind, Will began to see Gregg refracted through his new wife's eyes, and he started to come down way too hard on him. So Gregg was the black sheep at Will's house and the goat of his siblings at ours.

Still, he earned straight A's in school and he never got into trouble. We were close, and he and John got along well. John coached his Little League teams, and I went out to watch him every game. Will and I went to see the pediatrician, Dr. Kendig, together about our differing styles of discipline, though. He thought I was too soft on Gregg, and I considered Will way too harsh and hypercritical. I thought he over-focused on the minor problems, without giving fair attention to all the good things Gregg did.

57

In any case, the doctor calmed our bristles. "As long as both of you are consistent in your interactions with the children, and they're secure knowing what to expect from each of you, there's no need for you to come to a consensus on this." That was unlikely anyway.

Dr. Kendig didn't fare so well in our minds later that year. He sent Gregg to an allergist, thinking his bronchial coughs might be more related to allergens in the air than bronchitis. The tests—two series of fifty skin-pops on his back, terrifically painful—registered about eighty positive responses. Gregg would need allergy shots. Essentially, he was allergic to everything inside our house and everything outside it, too. We figured out the logistics: John would drive him into the doctor's office twice a week, after school. Eventually, this would devolve to once a week and lessen from there. This didn't work. Gregg was anxious the entire twenty-five-minute drive to the doctor. He'd beg John not to make him go. John hated it, so he gave Gregg a choice. Would he prefer John give him the shots at home, or did he want to keep getting them at the doctor's office? Gregg picked home, so John got the nurses to teach him how to give the shots. We put the medicine in our refrigerator, and John started injecting him. Gregg still hated the shots, but he took them with his usual stoicism since he didn't have all that buildup. This led to a sort of blow-up with Dr. Kendig.

He referred us to an otolaryngologist at MCV to check out Gregg's ears. This is normal procedure for a child with allergies, I understood. When we got there, the doctor took Gregg into an examining room, looked at him for no more than five minutes, closely scrutinizing each ear, then asked me to bring my child and come into his office. This was done so abruptly I followed along, no questions asked. He glanced at Gregg's chart, asked me the number at Dr. Kendig's office, then called him on the phone. In my presence, he told off Dr. Kendig.

"I've never seen a child's ears look like this. It looks like he has glue in them. Why did you wait so long to refer him?" I was stunned; if one doctor is going to call another doctor onto the carpet, don't they do it in private? After dispensing with his collegial upbraiding, the specialist explained to me that Gregg would need tubes in both ears, the sooner the better. He couldn't have been hearing well for some time. (This HAD to be related to his late talking, I'm sure, though the doctor didn't say so at the time.) The surgery itself was simple, a routine procedure, but the child had to be anesthetized. He'd have the hospital arrange it.

This had been too fast, too unexpected. Tubes are fairly common, I came to understand, but I'd never heard of this procedure. Gregg had the surgery, and afterward, he vomited for hours. He was a dishrag, in and out of sleep and throwing up the rest of the day. He was robust looking, sturdy and rosy and handsome. But it seemed like he had an inordinate number of health problems. The other children went to the doctor for no more than their routine check-ups, but something unexpected was always cropping up with him. Despite his allergies and related health problems, Gregg continued to be a star in sports and to excel in school.

About this time, I got a call from my mother at school one day saying that my older brother Jimmy was in the university hospital's mental ward in Charlottesville. She wondered if I'd visit him to see what was going on. I called his brand-new wife—they'd married only a few months before—and found out he'd started talking a few nights earlier and hadn't been able to stop. He'd sat up through the night, rambling on, until finally, she took him to the emergency room, and they'd admitted him as a psychiatric patient. I left school, met John, and headed for Charlottesville. Before I left, I arranged with my stepfather to meet the boys at the school bus and stay at our house with them until I got home.

When we got back from seeing Jimmy, I was a wreck. My "big brother," a Ph.D. candidate in civil engineering at U.Va., had been sitting in his bed picking at the covers, babbling about meaningless things like the food and his VMI ring and nothing else that I could grab hold of in any coherent way. I didn't know what was wrong with him, but I knew it was bad. On the drive back from Charlottesville, John and I tried to get our minds around it, but we were confused and scared. Both my parents were waiting and anxious to hear what we'd found out, but first they had to tell me about a little accident involving Gregg. My stepfather had been late getting to the bus stop; Gregg and Jaison had gotten off the bus by themselves and fooled around playing on the way to the house. They'd found a soda bottle and started throwing it against a pole. Gregg had cut one finger pretty badly. Jaison had the presence of mind to go to a neighbor's, who helped with the bleeding until Pawpie got there and took Gregg to the hospital. The upshot of it all was that Gregg had stitches—he'd cut off a pretty good chunk of the tip of one finger—and he was in considerable pain. The doctor was hoping he wouldn't need a skin graft.

The skin swelled around the stitches and his finger hurt for days. At first, he had to sleep with it propped up in the air, to lessen the blood flow and subsequent swelling. While I was home with him, my brother got out of the hospital and went to stay with my mother. Apparently, they'd given him enough medication to sedate him, and since he'd voluntarily signed himself in he could voluntarily sign himself out, A.M.A. (Against Medical Advice). Mother still had no idea what his diagnosis was, or if she did, she wasn't telling me. A few weeks later, I learned that the psychiatrists had asked for a family meeting before he checked out, but my mother didn't invite me. Her excuse, later, was that I "had too much on my plate at the time." In any case, Jimmy couldn't go back to his university responsibilities any time soon, and he didn't know if he wanted to return to his marriage or not. He would stay with my parents while he got extensive outpatient therapy, meeting with a psychologist at least two times a week. I had no idea, still, what his diagnosis was.

Within days my brother drove out to our house in Ashland and asked if he could stay with us. We said of course; no way would we turn away my brother, mental illness or not. The fact that we had three children, I worked full-time, and John and I were struggling financially didn't even factor into our decision. Besides, being around children might be good for Jimmy. He was Melanie's godfather, and they were both interested in science and things cerebral, so it would be a plus if they got to know one another better. He could spend time outside with the boys, too. He'd always been athletic, though not particularly competitive. This could have an upside for everyone.

It didn't work that way. The children were glad to have him there, but they kept their distance. One day, on his way to the doctor on the bus, some teenagers had taunted my brother, pointing and saying, "There's one of the funny ones." My grandmother would've said he just "didn't look right." In any case, my notion of my kids being good for him was unrealistic. He was sicker than I realized, but I still had no idea what the actual problem was. John would sit up with him; they'd drink beer and talk for hours, but John had no better handle on the psychiatric issues than I did. I was working days, doing school work nights, and attending the children's activities. I didn't ignore my brother. I just didn't have much time to spend with him.

His wife began to come over on the weekends. They didn't have much privacy in our house, so they'd take long walks in the woods behind us. She had a calming effect on Jimmy, and I was hopeful he'd get better. One sunny weekend, Gregg came hurtling into the house.

"Mama! Mama!" I could only imagine, *What now?* He ran up to me, but he was laughing, not crying. "Guess what, Mama," he yelled. Before I could say what he kept on. "I just saw Uncle Jimmy and Aunt Diana back in the woods . . . and they were naked!" What could I say? "Married people like to be naked together. It's okay." He ran off to tell Melanie and Jaison.

Not too much later, we heard Jaison up in the boys' loft one day after school. Gregg, seven years old and curious, had a little neighbor girl up there with him.

"Gregg, you better put your clothes on or you're gonna get in big trouble," Jaison screamed. When John came home they had "the talk." It was clearly time for it, though seven seemed young to both of us.

We went on vacation to the beach, thinking we could leave Jimmy at the house and he'd welcome the solitude. He'd been sending out resumés, looking for jobs, and he was seeing his doctor less. When we got back, though, he was morose. He apologized for not remembering my birthday, and I told him we'd just have to have a double celebration on his, twelve days after mine. But we never had that party. A few days later, John, the children, and I were at my mother's for dinner. Jimmy was late. The phone rang, and it was for me or John. I took it.

A policeman said, "Do you know a James D.?" I assured him I did, that he was my brother. He'd been found in his car in a wooded part of the county; he'd rigged up a hose from the exhaust. The car ran out of gas, so he was alive, but just barely. The ambulance had taken him to the emergency room at MCV. We should get there right away.

I had to tell my mother. She never changed her expression, just grabbed her purse. On the way to the hospital, my stepfather driving, she turned to me and asked, "Now tell me, Charlotte, what exactly is carbon monoxide poisoning?" She was no doubt in shock. When we got there I wouldn't let her go in to see him until after I did, and then I wouldn't let her go in at all.

When I called the psychologist to find out how my brother had reached such a desperate mental state, he told me that in his opinion Jimmy hadn't been suicidal. The absurdity of saying such a thing didn't get by me, but I didn't want to alienate this man. I wanted information from him. In all likelihood, it wouldn't help Jimmy now, but I had children. I knew mental illness had a strong familial component. I tried to stay calm. What HAD he been, then, if "not" suicidal? Suffering from depression, an anxiety disorder, and borderline personality disorder. Three diagnoses? His prognosis had been good, the doctor assured me. When I hung up, before I could explain my conversation to my parents—my mother was still thinking that a doctor could do something—I had to sit still for a few moments. My brother was dying, he'd tried to kill himself, but he hadn't been suicidal.

It took his brain three weeks to die. I was working at school that summer, in instructional planning, but I took emergency leave and went to the hospital to be with my brother every day. We told the children that Uncle Jimmy had been in a bad car accident, he was in the hospital dangerously sick, and they should say prayers for him. They went to their other parents, which felt natural enough to them, since they were scheduled to do that for part of the summer vacation anyway. I was the hospital liaison with the family, and they told me early on that despite his so-called alertness (wild eyes constantly jumping all over the place was alertness?) and his occasional ability to blurt out a word or two, the likelihood that he would recover was minuscule. If he lived, he'd be in a permanent vegetative state. He died the fifth of July, which was a blessing.

My parents decided on a graveside service, with only family. The children came home for that, dressed in Sunday clothes and looking strangely grownup. Melanie and Jaison cried and talked about Jimmy and tried to make their Nanny feel better; Gregg didn't. He'd made some drawings. Would we put them in Uncle Jimmy's casket so he could take them with him to Heaven? This surprised us. Jaison was our artistic child. John was blown away by Gregg's ink drawings; they looked like ancient religious iconography. Crosses but not crosses; circles with dark spaces inside, with zagged lines like bursts of energy shooting out. That boy never ceased to stun us; what was he thinking when he was so quiet so often? He was solemn during the service and stuck right by me, but he kept his sadness inside. This was the children's first experience with death, and I worried what impact it would have on all of them, since Uncle Jimmy had become part of their daily lives. John and I were ready to answer any questions, but none of them asked to talk much about it, and we didn't force them. We decided, too, they were all too young to know, at that time, that he'd attempted suicide.

That fall my friend Nancy died at home, as she wished, after her long, relentless struggle with cancer. For weeks she'd survived on pain killers, but her end was peaceful. She'd been a part of Melanie and Gregg's lives since they were born, and after John and I married, we all continued to go out to the farm to visit. Now she was dead, too, and we all mourned the loss of another member of our "big, real" family. The boys accepted it, but Melanie became despondent. I was fast to take her to a child psychologist. The cloud of my brother's illness hovered in the back of my mind, and I didn't want to miss any early signals if one of the children seemed uncommonly sad. The woman therapist we talked to saw Melanie once and assured us she was fine, just trying to deal with the loss of control in her world. She'd lost her family as she'd known it through divorce, her uncle, and now her lifelong adult friend and godmother. It was overwhelming, but she was healthy, not clinically depressed. I was relieved and glad for the reinforcement that other than predictable sadness at so many serious things she'd faced, she was okay.

When Melanie and Gregg went to Will's for their summer visit, an incident occurred that was disturbing, but since it was over when I found out, I filed it away as something to store should anything else happen. Apparently, Melanie and Nancy's son Matthew had been doing something together at the farm and Gregg was excluded. This was not unusual; they were both four years older than he was. At some point, Melanie taunted her brother about nobody wanting to play with him, and Will reported that Gregg flew into a scary rage and was beating Melanie without holding back any punches until Will had to pull Gregg off her. When Will eventually described this to me, he had dealt with it in terms of talking to Gregg and punishing him, but he was concerned about the extent of Gregg's anger. Our policy had been to each handle what occurred as soon as it occurred, and while I continued to look out for signs of Gregg being unduly angry in the months to come, or mean to his sister, I was not to see any evidence again for some time. I observed him, wondering if he might need to see a therapist, but he appeared happy. In fact, Melanie and Jaison got into some unpleasant arguments, but Gregg remained on the sidelines.

That spring, summer, and fall, some of the natural rhythm of our family life fell back into place, an enormous relief for all of us. All three children played recreational ball of one sort or another. We took our annual trip to Nags Head, and we went to Silver Bay on Lake George, a YMCA resort in the Adirondacks that the boys loved. They'd take sailing and play tennis and go on chaperoned overnights. It was a great place for all of us to heal. When school started in the fall, we all went back with renewed health and optimism.

By October, I had a big surprise for the children—for all of us. I was expecting a baby. A few years earlier I'd had a D & C for "female problems," and later I'd had a partial oophorectomy (ovary removal). I was approaching thirty-eight and hadn't expected to get pregnant. John and I were thrilled, and the boys responded with excitement. They couldn't wait until the baby's birth in April.

Melanie's response was unexpected. "Don't you dare get out of the car when you pick up carpool; I'd be mortified." Obstetrics had changed considerably since Gregg was born. I learned Lamaze, and my o.b. even told me the children could pack a snack and wait with me and John in the birthing room during labor and delivery. That was a bit TOO "modern" for all of us. After Miranda was born naturally, without complications, the boys came to the hospital to see her. Thirteen and ten, they were making all kinds of big brother plans. Melanie, almost fifteen, didn't come to see her new sister; she only insisted, "Don't expect me to change diapers or babysit. No way!"

We realized quickly enough that even happy changes in family dynamics create stresses. Our home in Ashland was twenty-five minutes away from the school where we both taught. Jaison was going to a private day school that would end in seventh grade; we'd be looking around for options for him, and there were none nearby at the time in Hanover County. Melanie was already enrolled in a private day school in Richmond, on the far west end away from the northside school where John and I both taught. We didn't have a nursery for the baby (our home had only three bedrooms; putting the baby in with Melanie was the only solution, but it was bound to create even more friction than she already felt about her "old" mother having another child). We had friends who ran a daycare center, but that was in a part of the county opposite the drive to Richmond. It was a logistical mess, and I suggested the only feasible solution: we needed to move to Richmond.

None of us, except Melanie, were big fans of the idea. We loved our home, the boys had friends and sports ties to the area, and our mortgage was low. We did it all the same, moving five minutes away from where John and I taught. Melanie's best friend Kara lived on the same block, another girl her age lived next door, and Kara's mom was willing to come babysit Miranda at our home while we worked. All in all, it was another positive change, but not without its sense of sadness and the usual moving tensions. Jaison never complained, and Gregg had nothing to say one way or the other. The faculty came over and helped us paint the big old three-story house, the children each had a private bedroom, and the baby had a nursery. Once we were settled all of us were glad we'd extended the effort. John and I worried about finances, especially with two children in private school and a baby requiring childcare, but we'd made it before and we'd make it again.

Gregg was the only child still in public school. In fifth grade by now, he went to a heavily integrated neighborhood elementary school, and he was perfectly happy there. He started taking his boombox and tapes to class, learning to do some of the inner city dances. The boys could ride their bikes around the neighborhood. After school and sports, they tended to do a lot together. Jaison often brought home friends from school, but Gregg almost never did. Gregg's happiness at that school was short-lived, though.

One day John got a call from the principal. Gregg was going to be suspended for a day, but first a parent had to come in for a conference. I was working, so without even telling me, John went. Gregg had kicked a hole in the boys' bathroom wall. No one was really sure why, not even his teacher. Gregg wouldn't talk to them about it, so they had no choice but to suspend him. John assured him we'd talk to Gregg and get to the bottom of it, and of course we'd expect to pay for the cost for repair.

As he was about to leave the office, the principal asked, "What do you think about Gregg's role in the play?" John, mystified, told him Gregg hadn't told us about any role or any play. Well, the fifth and sixth-grade classes were putting on a performance for the school for Martin Luther King, Jr. Day, and Gregg was scheduled to play James Earl Ray. John went ballistic, he told me later. Why would they portray that aspect of King's history in the first place? Why would they have one of the few white children in the class portray the assassin? The principal only shrugged, claiming it was up to the teachers. John made it clear that not only would Gregg NOT play Ray, he would not participate in the program, period.

At home, Gregg told me what had happened. Not his teacher, but one of the sixth-grade teachers, a large African-American woman, "teased" him often when she saw him. He claimed she'd say things like, "Just wait'll I get you in my class next year, little white boy. You won't be such a smart bigshot then." Always smiling, but it upset him. He knew our family was totally pro-civil rights. He didn't want to cause a big stir, but she made him uncomfortable. That day in the auditorium, he'd sat kicking the back of the seat in front of him, a nervous habit he had, even in the car. She came up the aisle and told him to stop, and he did. After that, he started tapping the arms of his chair with his wrists; he swore he wasn't making any noise or talking. He was watching the rehearsal. Again she came up to him, and this time she yelled. "You better stop that knocking or you're gonna be sorry." He said his eyes started watering—she was large, she scared him, and her voice was angry—and then with hands on hips, she yelled at him in front of everyone. "So the little white boy's a sissy. He's gonna cry. You better go to the bathroom and wash your face, little white boy, if you're gonna cry like a girl." That's when he'd gone to the boys' room and kicked a hole in the wall.

John reported this all back to the principal the next day, who revealed that this teacher had been moved from another school for this very kind of behavior, but Gregg would have to fulfill his suspension just the same. We started procedures for him to change schools to go to a private boys' school in the city. He would be far better off there, intellectually and academically, and perhaps he'd also have the chance to shine in sports. The financial bucket was empty, our budget was a disaster, but we felt like we had no choice. Gregg transferred that fall. Another change in a string of changes.

CHAPTER 5 – WE BOTH WOBBLE

Gregg's entry into private school life started off mostly well. He was a standout in sports from the first. His grades remained high. He was able to take new-to-him classes like Latin, which he loved from the beginning. The boys played some academic form of baseball with roots and word parts and they got into it; it was a chance for Gregg to shine. Plus the Latin teacher was also the weight-training coach, and in seventh grade, Gregg started lifting when he could. There was a lot he liked about his new school, and for the first time, he began making friends he enjoyed and bringing them home. One had his same offbeat sense of humor, another was the jock type, and both thought Gregg was great. We were pleased with his choices and delighted we'd made the school change.

We'd encouraged Gregg to take Boys' Choir, though, and this did not work well. He loved to sing, but this group was regimented, serious, and demanding. He thought it would be fun. He started to show up at performances late, without his music, or in wrinkled white shirts or khakis, because he hadn't given me enough warning that he needed them. The director urged him to stay in the group but told him he'd have to shape up. He decided to quit. I didn't mind, thinking he'd given it a try, and he was adjusting to a new, more rigorous environment. His time was already pretty stretched with academic and sports demands.

Signs of anger or mental problems? Not during this period. Those three accounts of undue anger—the one by his pre-school teacher, the fight with his sister, the teacher incident—struck me as far apart, unrelated, and not signals of some deep, ongoing problem. Everyone who met Gregg said, "What a great kid!" One family we saw year after year at the beach; their daughter, Theresa, an only child, was a little younger than Gregg. We grown-ups always sat on the beach and talked while the children played. Theresa and her parents would take both boys for ice cream in the evenings and come back talking about how great they both were— about how "dreamy" Theresa found Gregg. With his hazel-green eyes, his muscular build, and his quiet "sweet" manners (their words, not mine), they found him a "pleasure" to be around. One summer on the beach, the dad challenged the boys to see how long they could hit the beach paddle ball between them without missing. Gregg and Jaison and the dad set the goal at something ridiculous, like five hundred; they didn't miss until they got to a thousand, when they stopped. Finally, both boys had their feet on the ground, or so we thought.

At Silver Bay, when Gregg was about thirteen, John and Gregg entered the father/son doubles tennis tournament. No one thought they had a chance; one of the families had a long tennis tradition there, and Gregg was a relative "newbie," not only at camp but to tennis. His sports were football, basketball, and baseball, but he had the natural grace and agility as well as the needed mental strategizing skill for tennis, too, even though he wasn't very experienced. When John and Gregg won that year, I've never seen two bigger smiles.

Gregg went to UVA basketball camp that summer, also. He was short—even as an adult he never grew beyond five-ten—

which annoyed him to no end. In our family, that wasn't a shrimp boat, since none of us is what you'd describe as tall, but in most sports, he was deemed too small to be considered much of a college scholarship contender. Still, he was an excellent point guard; his ball-handling, quickness, and play-making stood him in good stead, despite his height. When we sent him to basketball camp for a week, we wondered how he'd do against the far bigger boys from across the state and even East Coast. When we went to pick him up, he was sitting on a hill in front of his dorm, surrounded by five trophies. As the successes piled up, I felt that he was certainly past the "trauma" of his parents divorcing and remarrying, and the only way for him now was up.

He was all boy, but when he came home from school each day, he'd run to Miranda's room and sing to her. "Hush little baby, don't say a word," he'd croon as he rubbed her back. Melanie, of course, didn't want to be "tied" to babysitting; Jaison was a social gadabout. Perhaps it was the fact that Gregg was the youngest of the older three, but as much as the other two adored Miranda, they had too many teenage activities going on at that period of their lives to spend much time with her. Gregg was the one who volunteered to read to her or pull her in her wagon or teach her songs. Sunday nights we'd make sourdough bread together. He loved doing this, and we'd get to talk about school and sports and books, a rare time alone in our boisterous household.

Of course, as Gregg got more into that adolescent mindset, he changed, too. When I went back to grad school at night and the three of them were home with their precocious little sister (John often had to teach nights at the Virginia Museum; we needed his second job more than ever), I often came back to a surprise.

One night toddler Miranda greeted me with her middle finger held up. "Hi, Mama!" she beamed. Jaison and Gregg were doubled over laughing. Their baby sister was in the dark.

"What have you two taught her?" I demanded.

71

She kept on shaking her middle finger saying "Hi, Hi, H'lo." They'd told her that sticking up "tall man" was a friendly way to say hi, like waving.

Another time, she was running around the house saying "Damn! Damn! Damn!"

"Okay, guys. I know you did this!" I confronted the boys. Of course. They'd taught her damn meant the same as phooey or too bad or some other acceptable way of complaining. But since they laughed every time she said it, she said it continuously.

Their TV viewing was limited to an hour a night, and they had to agree on what they'd watch. Since the three older ones rarely agreed on anything, which was no surprise, they rarely watched television. During the first Iraq War, though, they would have assignments to keep up with the news, and they all had permission to do their required viewing. I avoided having Miranda in the room, but I never worried that perhaps absorbing images of the bombings and destruction was "too much information" for Gregg at his age.

At Melanie's request (more like begging night and day), we took in a boarder who she'd spent two summers with at Nature Camp. Both of them were juniors; Robin's mother wanted her to go to private school, but in their rural part of western Virginia there wasn't an option. I wanted an open home. The family only paid me $50 a month for the girl's board, and that was sometimes late coming, but my idea was if we had the room, why not give a hand up? Robin came to live with us, she attended the same school Melanie attended, and what was one more plate at the table? They didn't send a car with her, so she depended on Melanie or other friends to get around, but I wasn't too concerned. She was a lovely, personable gal; she was into art and the school had an excellent art program, and the boys didn't mind having her around at all (she was "easy on the eyes" as my grandmother might have said). The second year she lived with us, her senior year, she and Melanie didn't get along that well any longer, she wrecked our family car (an in-city accident that was not her fault), and with Gregg a high school freshman and Jaison a junior, we got spread too thin all around, but I wouldn't go back on my commitment, and we made it work, like any family would.

The summer between middle school and high school, Gregg was invited to the beach, on a chaperoned trip with a group of the boys and parents. We were delighted. It turned into a nightmare, though, when we found out he'd gotten into trouble for drinking. He wasn't the only one, but he got caught, sent home, and we grounded him. As shocked and upset as we were, we speculated that him "getting nailed" was probably a good thing. We knew we could count on the chaperones, he knew we weren't going to put up with underage drinking, and he'd gotten out of the experience safe and whole—sick as a whipped dog, but safe. Perhaps we could breathe a bit easier knowing that he'd passed that marker and learned the boundaries. Rumors about private school drinking abounded in our region, and all in all, we'd landed well. If Melanie and Jaison were drinking, we didn't know about it.

Gregg and Jaison went to different private schools; Gregg needed Latin and Advanced Math, while Jaison's mom wanted him to go to a military prep school. They didn't get to attend one another's sporting events or hang out with the same guys, so naturally, they didn't get to do as many things together as they once had, except our annual beach vacations. This was too bad, since when they were home they got along so well. If they complained to anyone they complained to one another; I never heard either of them grouse about much. Maybe a car, maybe curfew extensions, but neither of them was a complainer. Jaison didn't get bad behavior reports any more at all, and in middle school, neither did Gregg.

As a freshman, Gregg made two of the three varsity sports, which made us proud but ended up causing headaches. As he hung out with the older boys, he became not only quiet but secretive. I didn't know how to tease out what was a teenage turning point and

73

what should be cause for concern. But quite frankly, as long as he wasn't getting in trouble, I wasn't digging too deeply. With four teenagers and a toddler in the house, a full-time teaching job, and a husband out a couple of evenings a week working, I was juggling as fast as I could.

Melanie graduated and we had a lovely party. The pictures are beautiful—her in a beautiful white dress holding roses, beaming; Gregg and his two stepbrothers in coats and ties smiling; Will and Betti and my family all around a celebration table together. We looked like a happy, proud blended family that night. I am certain we were.

That summer, just before his freshman year, at Silver Bay, Gregg got into some serious trouble. The YMCA program runs dry campuses for its resorts. This had never been a problem. We learned, to our surprise, that the teenagers who knew one another well from years of coming to family week together often went off campus at night, and part of their partying involved drinking, lots of drinking. This would have been disturbing enough, because of the dangers of driving those twisting mountainous roads, but this particular night when we found all this out, Gregg was not only drinking. He got into a fight with another camper and broke his nose. He had to confront some of the other dads and apologize, and we had to face the fact that his secretive drinking was becoming a serious problem. John talked to him, his dad talked to him; we grounded him, he complied. Still, his quietness was disturbing. He didn't even try to argue or convince us what he did wasn't "all that bad," like any of the other three would have. He did what we said, but without apparent anger or shame or any seeming remorse.

I was Head of Instruction and Head of English by this time, both enormous responsibilities in our college prep school. That fall I coached drama as well. I'd written and directed the play, and by the time it was over, I was whipped. Just meeting my daily responsibilities had become overwhelming, and I'd caught a cold I couldn't shake. The night the play closed and we had the cast party at school, I crawled into bed, put my head on the pillow exhausted, and the phone rang. It was the campus police at the local university. John answered; someone needed to come and pick up Gregg. He'd been caught in a car full of guys drinking a six-pack. Clearly intoxicated, he'd been mouthy to the policeman, too, and he was banned from the campus. They'd hold him until a parent arrived. John went for him and I called his dad. We had a crisis on our hands, no ifs, ands, or buts. Gregg was grounded again except for school activities. All the parents united on this. Of course he was mad at us, but that didn't matter. He needed to understand that we weren't going to look the other way while he drank. One way or the other we'd stop it.

In the upper school, he started having other disturbing problems, also. He got in trouble when he talked to his history teacher in inappropriate ways. He claimed the guy insulted his buddies in his classes, and when the instructor said something Gregg deemed demeaning to one of his friends, Gregg insisted he had to take up for his pal, which involved impertinence. But then his English teacher reported that Gregg made an off-the-wall sexual remark about the teacher and his girlfriend, some aside in the hall completely out of line like "You get any this weekend?" All four parents and the school agreed he needed to "talk to" someone. The guidance counselor recommended a psychologist nearby who worked with their students; he could walk to the sessions during school hours and they'd schedule around it.

When he had his initial psychological testing, he was "off the charts" in anger. (That word anger again; I couldn't help but feel frightened now—and emotionally responsible for failing to believe it way back when and getting help earlier.) All other measures and indicators of problems fell within normal range. But the anger was a huge red flag. Gregg started going to the therapist, but reluctantly. He'd dawdle on the way, he complained about talking to a woman, he wouldn't open up. The heart of the problem finally had a name, we could see a focused way forward, but there's a world of difference between identification and solution, as we found out the hard way.

When I went to the doctor myself because of my continuing cough and relentless exhaustion, he advised medication and vitamins, but he also thought I should see a psychologist. I was ready to listen; I wanted and needed help.

I did get back into therapy again, this time on my own, this time willingly. I found a psychologist who came highly recommended by the group I'd taken Melanie to see when Nancy died. I liked their cognitive rather than Freudian approach. I wasn't trying to dig up any sins of the past, mine or anyone else's. I wanted to get a handle on my complicated life and figure out why I was tired all the time. After the first session, including a standard questionnaire, Dr. Marilyn Spiro determined I was clinically depressed and probably had been for some time. She started me on a regimen of Prozac, and we set up regular weekly appointments. Gregg and I were both getting help; this had to be an upswing, a shift toward the right direction.

John and I decided to take all the children to Disney World for Christmas. Miranda at five was at a fun age for that, and with Melanie in college, the time to do it was slipping away. Besides, sitting on the beach in the sun sounded like a tonic to me. All of the children loved the water and would surely enjoy the beach in winter. A friend of ours had a cottage in the Tampa/St. Pete area, right on the ocean that we could rent inexpensively. Melanie, a college freshman, surely wouldn't mind getting a tan over Christmas. We all did better when we had some space to get away from one another and some physical activity. I got the okay from Will, but unfortunately, Jaison's mom said no. The five of us would drive down, then, the three adults taking turns with the driving, and we'd go to Disney World one day with Miranda. The rest of the time we'd relax, soak up some rays, and take long walks on the beach. Only that was the year Florida had its hundred-year snowstorm.

It was cold, and our cottage wasn't geared for the cold. That was okay; we had blankets and sweatshirts. We couldn't cook on the electric stove because the power was on and off. No problem; we could go out to eat. That first night set the unfortunate tone for the entire week: one child wanted seafood, another wanted pizza, and Miranda was so hungry and fussy that we finally went to the first place that had electricity, which nobody liked. This was not going well. We couldn't go out on the beach while it was snowing. This was a wet, blowing snow. We were closed up in the house and started to get on one another's nerves big time.

The next day, ice was falling. John took Gregg and Melanie with him to pick oranges and grapefruits at our friends' place. The night temperature was going down to freezing, the fruit would be destroyed, so they had to get it all boxed and in the garage before dark. I was too tired to help. That evening the city had brown-outs; it alternated power times between quadrants of the city, and we tried to stay warm and use candles to read. Television wasn't an option, since it was an extraneous use of power and we were supposed to ration, turning on lights during our "brown" phases only for essentials. The next day, the teenagers were bored, I was grouchy, and Miranda wanted someone to play with, but no one was in a playing mood. We sent the older two to scout for a take-out pizza, mostly to get them out of our hair. I remember wanting to sleep, and to sleep deeply enough so I wouldn't have to deal with my family's needs or this horrid vacation. I went into the bathroom to get a Tylenol. I didn't intend to take more than two. But I did. I never had a single thought of suicide. After I swallowed every one of a new large bottle, I went into the bedroom to lie down. All I remember is closing my eyes and thinking, *Ah, this is so peaceful. I'll finally get some rest.* I was tired, I was tired, I was tired . . .

Apparently, John found the empty bottle in the bathroom, got me up, and we had a scene in front of Miranda. He wanted to call the hospital, I refused to let him, and we pulled the telephone back and forth until we pulled it out of the wall. Needless to say, this was off the charts for us—I didn't usually raise my voice, and here I was raging in front of my husband and child. When Melanie and Gregg walked in the door with the pizza, the ambulance and the police were there. Somehow our friends had arrived, too. I had no choice; I went to the emergency room.

When I next saw my family standing over me in the E.R., I remember Gregg looking down at me with sad, frightened eyes. He was on my left side, holding my hand. John was on the right. Melanie was at my feet, looking mad and confused. Why had I done this horrible thing? I had no rational answer for them; I'd only intended to take a couple of aspirin, take a nap. Dazed and weak—how had this happened?—I told them all I loved them, that I never wanted to leave them.

Gregg held onto my hand and said, "I love you too, Mom. Please be all right." He was near tears. John and Gregg kissed me, they left, and I slept.

A young handsome psychiatrist interviewed me in the morning. I sat up, he asked me questions, I answered. "Had I had hallucinations prior to taking the Tylenol? For example, did voices tell me to take them?"

"Of course not."

"Any delusions, like I could fly?"

"What? Never. NO!" On and on. Did he think I was nuts? I explained, "I was exhausted. I wanted to sleep. For some irrational reason, I looked at myself in the mirror and downed the whole bottle. I had NO prior intention to 'do something' to myself. I needed a nap."

"Did I think at that moment that I wanted to die?"

"Ridiculous! I'm scared to death of dying. I love my husband. I love my children. I don't want to die!" I'd come mighty close, though, he told me. He had a medical explanation for my actions, which I clung to but no one else seemed to believe: a rare reaction to my anti-depressant. I refused to think that I was a crazy person; except for that one insane thing I'd done, I didn't feel like an insane person. He said, quite simply, that my dose of Prozac was too low. He explained that one of the uncommon reactions to beginning users is impulsive irrational behavior. He tripled my dosage, called my prescribing psychiatrist in Virginia, and allowed me to leave with John and the children that afternoon. Each of them viewed me with suspicious eyes. John was scared and angry; Melanie was just plain angry. Gregg was sad and guilty—and quiet. Miranda was whimpery and clingy. I had brought this on my family, the people I loved most in the world. I had no right to bring such turmoil and pain into my home, I was clear about that, but I'd done it.

Christmas was the next day. Our friends had us over for dinner. We exchanged gifts and put forth the effort to be cheerful for Miranda, but everyone was on edge. The cold weather hadn't let up, and though it wasn't snowing, we still could barely go outside. I sat on the beach and played Trivial Pursuit with Melanie and Gregg later in the day, in the wintry sunlight, hoping for some semblance of relaxation. No one talked about the obvious topic; Melanie got furious if anybody brought it up. We all tried to "carry on." That night, John caught Gregg smoking. On the scale of the current crisis, it hardly raised a blip, but we hated it. He knew better. We all knew better.

When we got home—a terrible drive, with seething college freshman Melanie blowing up and yelling awful things at me in a restaurant. Her unleashed anger infuriated John, but I couldn't blame her, she had every right to be furious. I was relieved to be in my own bed again, didn't want to argue any more. Sick as I felt, I was far more pained in my heart over the trauma I'd caused John and the children. Melanie and Gregg went to Will's for the remainder of the school holiday; John must have asked them to keep all this to themselves for the time being, but I don't remember that. For once he was making unilateral decisions, and I didn't care. He and I were tiptoeing around one another, each trying to avoid any kind of upsetting outburst, both holding knots of fear and feelings locked inside. I talked to my psychologist on the telephone. She strongly advised that I check into a women's treatment program for at least thirty days.

"That's impossible!" was my initial reaction. John assured me it was possible. I needed it; we'd make it work. But what about my teaching job, Miranda, the busy-ness of our lives? Who'd manage? We made the arrangements, and John and Miranda took me to the Psychiatric Institute of Richmond that same night.

John promised, "I'll take charge of everything." Once he kissed me goodbye, I wasn't to worry about the children or the job or the bills. I was to work on getting well. Confused myself and uncertain why I was there—what exactly did that mean, "getting well"?—I went through the check-in process. My iron was low, my red blood cells were low, my white blood cells were low, I couldn't have had any energy or any resistance. Still, that wasn't the "presenting problem." I was clinically, chronically depressed—had been for years, from my history. The intake nurse explained about showers and sharps and schedules and took me to my room, more like a college dorm room than any hospital room I'd ever seen. Though two beds were made up, I didn't have a roommate. That night they assigned me an aide, and I was to be checked every fifteen minutes. Didn't anybody get it? I didn't want to kill myself. The one thing I needed was rest, and it looked like I wouldn't get that here, either.

My psychiatrist saw me the next morning. I loved him, Dr. David Markowitz. Though he wasn't my psychologist, whenever I saw him, he always talked with me for ten minutes or so about what was going on. He wasn't so quick to dismiss the suicide attempt as an adverse reaction to the medication. People had unconscious desires, he reminded me. I didn't like that one bit and told him so; or maybe I just think I told him so. At that point, I was still trying to be the good girl and the good patient, to make him admire me as the best depressed person he'd ever treated. My brother had committed suicide. I hated suicide. Nancy and I had talked about it, when she was in so much pain the last six months of her life, when she couldn't even read because the cancer in her brain had blurred her vision.

She told me, "You know, I contemplated it, taking an overdose, when things got real bad. But after I saw what Jimmy's death did to you and your family, I knew I could never do it. I couldn't do that to Matthew and Andy. It's the selfish way out." I agreed with that. I'd never fantasized about suicide myself. I was just exhausted from dealing with never-ending demands and problems.

Dr. Marcowitz looked at my bloodwork. I needed vitamins and iron. He'd oversee the new dosage of Prozac, too. This was the right step in my treatment. But medicine alone wasn't going to bring about a "cure," he insisted. I needed to work with the program.

When my psychologist, Marilyn Spiro, came to see me, I nearly cried. She was my lifeline. As she told me early in our work together, she had an excellent bullshit detector, and she wasn't about to let me get away with any phony crap. Her baseline question was always, "What do you want right now?" That morning, she didn't need to linger over whether my overdose was intentional or not. How was I dealing with it? What did I want to do about it? What did I want to gain, now that the bus had stopped and let me off and I had the chance to deal with MY problems for a change? I wanted to know, first and foremost, how to put things right with my children. That would and could wait, she insisted. I had to work on me.

I would take groups every day in the program called "Escape to Reality." A Women's Issues Group, a Co-Dependence group, and an exercise group. Plus therapy. The best thing I could do was dive in and be honest. For a while, she'd see me daily, too, but that would taper off. The group leaders were all psychologists themselves, and women, except for the exercise leader. He was a man, and the founding psychiatrist of the women's program. It struck me as odd that he taught the exercise class, but what about this whole experience wasn't odd?

Every morning all the women gathered. A daily quote appeared on the chalkboard (from an affirmation book, I came to know). We were to welcome any new women into the circle and talk about the quote. Sort of like what I'd heard AA to be like, or prison groups. The patients varied in age from late teens to seniors. My age group, late thirties, early forties, was well represented. A nurse sat in with us, most everyone said something predictable, like "My husband is mean to me" or "I hate my mother," and we went to a cafeteria area for breakfast. The facility was clean, the women didn't appear "crazy," as I'd feared, drooling or babbling and wandering about like in *The Snake Pit* or *One Flew Over the Cuckoo's Nest*. They looked no crazier than I felt, which I found ironic. Here we all were. I wondered why.

I held onto my "Nothing's really wrong with me, I need a rest" façade for a long time. Too long. Meanwhile, one of the most attractive women on the hall, a bright mother of two, revealed she was physically abused by her husband but still loved him, couldn't leave him. Another older woman, with grown children, had tried to leave her husband. He'd put a gun to her head. When she'd told him to go ahead and shoot, he didn't. A drop-dead gorgeous Black woman had a shopping obsession; she'd ruined her family financially and still couldn't stop. Her therapist uncovered childhood sexual abuse by her cousins. One's husband was selling "crank" (Did she mean crack? No. Crank) out of their garage. They had more money than you could fit into a Brink's truck; she was constantly afraid for her safety and that of her children. If the Feds didn't get them, the drug lords would. Was she making all this up? Okay, I was depressed. That was nothing like these problems, though. I could take a pill and be better, return to my demanding life and manage it. I went through group after group after group, especially my codependence group, without scratching the surface of my deep depression.

John visited daily. He didn't flicker in his devotion. I allowed certain other close friends to come, but I refused to talk to my birth family, except for my younger brother Victor, a Vietnam vet who kept his distance from our family, who called from Panama. His unexpected "Are you okay?" lifted me. Who knew he cared? Jaison came to see me one day, still in his school uniform.

He turned the radio on and said, "Come on, Charlotte, let's dance." As we did, he told me, tears welling, "I always thought you were perfect." My heart broke right then, at both his tenderness and his love for me. Gregg came a number of times. The first few times he was sweet, too. The last time he had to tell me he'd gotten in trouble again. At a party. Drinking involved. Some girl he'd gone upstairs with. They'd fooled around but hadn't had sex. Now she was telling all their friends he'd tried to rape her. I made him look me in the eye: Had he? He swore no. All the times he'd been in trouble he'd never lied when caught. Sometimes he'd even confessed before he was caught. I had to believe him this time. Besides, I was in the looney bin; I wasn't supposed to be dealing with family trauma like this. I made him promise he'd tell his father and his therapist. John and I couldn't handle this crisis this time. We were dealing with way more than we could manage already. Oddly, nothing ever came of it—maybe this girl was gossiping in such a sadistic way?—but it was one more worry about Gregg that nagged.

Psychiatric Institute of Richmond was an amazing program. By the end, I'd "given up" my desperate hold on my chronic depression and come to terms with the fact that I didn't know how to be happy and to "ask for what I needed." I'd bluffed my way through my own life, seemingly nonplussed by my parents' divorce, my mother's absence from our home while she worked two jobs and my grandmother raised us, her re-marriage, my father's subsequent move to Arizona when I was only eight (I saw him two more times in my life, once at my brother's college graduation; he died when I was 23), the loss of my grandmother when she moved out and took my younger brother with her. None of these things had bothered me, tra la—I hadn't even cried—because I'd made myself emotionally detached from my life. I'd smiled and succeeded in school. When my own first marriage wasn't working, instead of looking inward, I'd ended it. That's how I'd forbidden all that pain to hurt me, by detaching from it. But by closing out pain, I'd closed out all other emotions, too. Now I had to figure out how to be good to myself; only then could I be good to others, and adult in relationships. For the first time in my life, I got it; I felt it.

My new self-awareness was hardly a remedy for all the broken lives around me, though, for all the trouble I caused when I'd "lost it" in Florida. My doctors called a family get-together to allow my husband and children to say how they felt about all this and to come to grips with changes I needed to make when I came home. Jaison and Gregg had little to say, except they loved me. Miranda wanted me to come home. John understood, but couldn't believe I'd been unhappy inside that long.

Melanie was furious. "I drove here from UVA to hear this crap? You're depressed and unhappy? Well tough shit. You're the mom. Moms are supposed to get it together and take care of their kids." As far as she was concerned, I'd behaved terribly, and she hated me, and she didn't want to talk to me or anyone else about this ever again. She stormed out of the conference room. I was in tears. I understood it was healthy for her to express her anger. But I was too raw to have it directed at me with such force. I wasn't ready to go home. How could I pick up where I'd left off with Jaison and Gregg and Miranda? How would John deal with all this? When would I be able to talk to Melanie again, to try to patch our relationship? The family meeting had been a disaster, and I was still in the hospital. What in the world would it be like when I got home?

CHAPTER 6 -- SERIOUS TROUBLES

When I came home, I was resolved to focus on my own needs as I attended to my husband and children with as much love but less anxiety (or control) than before. I was working toward an M.F.A. in creative writing. I'd always loved to write, been recognized for my expressive ability throughout high school and college, but I'd never given myself "permission" to focus on that talent as a "real writer." As a child, one of my prized possessions had been my Tom Thumb typewriter; I'd written a neighborhood gossip rag on it, *The Giddy Girls' Club Gazette*, when I was around eight. I'd been an editor on the high school, award-winning newspaper, an English major in college. Reading and writing were two of my loves, but I made little time for them. One of the decisions I'd made in the hospital was to go back to grad school full-time for my final year, beginning that fall. That would give me a chance to finish my current professional obligations. It would also put a major economic strain on our family, but I needed to put writing more at the center of my life, and this would be a crucial beginning step.

John and I went out to a romantic dinner at one of our favorite Fan restaurants. "I'm going to stop working for a year and go to VCU full-time in the fall." I'd learned to make "I statements" in the hospital. For the first time, John faltered. How would we make it? We would, I promised. I'd apply for an internship; that would pay for my classes and give me a $7,000 stipend. The lines on his face, some from his worry over the last month, some from my unexpected decision, didn't diminish.

"Charlotte, I'll do whatever you want and need. But I don't see how this'll work." Our dinner out wasn't much of a celebration, but for once I didn't waver.

Melanie, away at school, continued to give me the cold shoulder. Jaison was playing varsity soccer and wasn't home much. Miranda was overjoyed to have me back home. She quickly backed off her clinginess and became her jolly affectionate self.

Though at night she'd call in from her bedroom next to ours, "You okay, Momma? You okay, Daddy?" Gregg, as unflappable as he was at home, continued to have minor problems at school. But he starred in sports. We changed his therapist, to a male psychologist noted for his work with adolescents. Since this man ran marathons, I was optimistic that the athletic connection would create an opening between him and Gregg. We thought perhaps he'd get beneath Gregg's stoic surface and help him.

Meanwhile, Gregg started dating a lovely young woman, Lara. Oddly enough, she went to the school where John and I taught, and we couldn't have been more pleased with his choice. At first, since he wasn't yet driving even though he was sixteen—the Morgan family could hardly afford a car per person—we'd drive him way across town to go to her house, and then we'd drive back at eleven to pick him up. They'd go to her choir practice and to Young Life together. Her family was quite religious. I'd "fallen away" from church after my divorce, but Will continued to take both children to services and Sunday School when they were with him, so I was pleased that Gregg was going out with a gal who didn't drink and who didn't need to party to have a good time. When Gregg got his license, we were doubly delighted. As we had with Melanie and Jaison, we gave him our "clunker" of a car instead of buying him one, and I bought the "new" used car for myself. Melanie had an old Datsun, which lasted her all through college. Jaison had the "Green Hornet," a Ford Fairmont station wagon. We gave Gregg my Honda Civic hatchback, clearly a "cooler" car than the other two had received, but still an older model with lots of mileage. For the first time, John had purchased a brand new Honda Accord off the lot for us. He loved that car.

One night when Lara was visiting at our house, we'd gone to bed early. Gregg was going to drive her home. This was a big relief, as we could go on upstairs and read and not worry about the cross-town round trip. Only, for some unknown reason, Gregg took the keys to the new car instead of taking his own car—one of his many spontaneous bad decisions, but the next one was worse. Going through the residential section, he wanted to show his gal how people "jumped" the speed bumps. But he crashed our car into the wooden railings in the median. Lara wasn't hurt, and neither was Gregg, but he panicked when he saw the damage to the car. He ran from the scene to tell us—poor judgment on his part, added to the poor judgment of speeding in the neighborhood, on top of the poor judgment of taking the new car instead of his own. The police became involved. John was beyond furious. Me? I was overwhelmed.

We made Gregg work to pay for his ticket and the city's cost of damages and the repairs to our new car—more than a thousand dollars. Usually, Gregg didn't cross us, verbally, but oddly enough, despite the obvious mistakes and responsibility on his part, this time he did. For the first time ever, he insisted that our consequences were unjust.

"That's what car insurance is for," he ranted, "to pay for accidents. This was an accident." We explained that this so-called accident occurred because of a bad decision on his part, that the rates for adolescent boys were off the charts, that even now with his good grade bonus our insurance would go sky high because of his reckless driving ticket, and it was only right that he pay for the repairs, since he'd taken the car without permission. He sulked and complained about this, but we didn't relent. This confrontational attitude over the wreck was the first time we'd experienced the kind of "you're being unfair to me" attitude at home that teachers had sometimes complained about at school in recent months.

This accident was the beginning of more serious troubles, too. That fall, still in counseling, Gregg fell asleep at the wheel, on the way home from a school event.

The officer called. "Are you Gregg Smith's mother?" Gregg was drunk, but he wouldn't get a ticket. Oh dear God; the policeman said that since the ignition was off, he couldn't ticket Gregg for drunk driving. Drunk AND driving? We'd missed his drinking altogether, again, thinking that he wasn't involved in that scene since Lara wasn't. The therapy clearly wasn't helping, but we all met together with the psychologist to "process" these events and pressed on. Lara stuck by him—I have no idea why—and we kept Gregg at home as much as we could. He stayed in his room a lot; he wasn't up in our faces complaining, and if he was brooding, he wasn't talking about it.

In the spring, I was scheduled to do a workshop in another city for a professional in-service program. I was getting my final notes and handouts together; Gregg had been at his dad's for the weekend. He'd gone on some school trip or sports activity. But instead of being where he was supposed to be that weekend, he'd gotten roaring drunk with his buddies. We found out that the guys had some abandoned school bus that they climbed into where they "slept it off," each claiming to be staying over at the other's house. Supposedly, that's what Gregg had done with his dad. Only sometime during the night he'd wandered into a nearby house, gone upstairs, and blacked out on a bed. When the woman who lived there got up on Sunday, she found him there, in her guest room, still passed out. She didn't call the police; I had no idea why.

I went to pieces. This was beyond any adolescent boy misbehavior I could put in some category of "rebelling" or "challenging authority." This was scary and dangerous and off the charts disturbing. To add to the bizarreness, the woman was the secretary at the private school Gregg attended. She'd recognized him and knew to call his dad. While he wouldn't be arrested, he was clearly in grave trouble. I canceled my speaking engagement, for once too upset to soldier on, knowing that it was going to be necessary to find some other way to help Gregg, and to find it fast. When I tried to talk to Gregg, he just shrugged and contended it was "no big," that the drinking himself into blackouts wasn't something for me to get so upset about. All his buddies did it. He wouldn't discuss it.

His dad and I blew apart on this one. I wanted Gregg to get more treatment—even different treatment, if we could figure out what that should be. But no, I did not want to ban him from his excellent school opportunity or playing sports. To my mind, this was the one "lifeline" he had, the only aspect of his life he could feel confident about. Plus it was healthy, a physical outlet. Stopping sports felt like a bad idea to me, counterintuitive, counter productive. True, we had to come up with a different approach: the counseling was a flop, Gregg was way out of control. I was willing to accede to that and look around to find the "different" thing that might help him, but I did not want him to change schools or give up sports. Neither did the head of his school, even in the face of this last fiasco. Gregg was smart, and this school was the right fit for his intelligence. The faculty knew him and were willing to work with him. I wanted him to stay put and find a better treatment fit.

Will and his wife came to my home one day; we'd scheduled a "sit down" to talk about Gregg and what we should all do to help him. John wasn't there, for some reason. I'm sure he was teaching or coaching. In any case, that session was the end of my ability to work affably and positively with Melanie and Gregg's father.

Betti told me, "You know, this all comes down to you being a bad mother. You must know that neither of your children even like you, and if you have any thought whatsoever for Gregg's well-being, you'll let him come and live with us." This was the proverbial sucker punch, right in the gut of my own self-doubt. I was stunned, speechless, shocked.

"A bad mother?" Will backed her up: If they had to, they'd fight me for custody. Approached in a different way, I might have viewed moving to his dad's as one of the possibilities I'd consider. Consider. Maligned, threatened, knowing that Gregg would only hate his father's rigid disapproval and his stepmother's disdain on a daily basis, I dug in my heels.

Literally. I walked all the way from my northside house to Willow Lawn that afternoon, unable to stay in the living room where that poisonous conversation occurred. My haven was fouled. An hour, an hour and a half later, I had to call John from a payphone to get him to pick me up.

I hired a lawyer. He assured me nothing I'd done would disqualify me as Gregg's custodial parent. Instead of allies, Will and I were now outspoken enemies. He'd call on the phone and berate me for "causing all this with the kids" and "ignoring my parental responsibilities." I'd cry for days. That was an unfortunate turning point for all of us, but especially for Gregg. Upset as I was, I sat him down eventually and offered the possibility of going to live with his dad. He swore he'd do anything except that. Having experienced Betti's attack side up close and personal, I didn't encourage it or bring it up again.

Without any dissension, Will and I did agree that Gregg required immediate, intensive treatment. Weekly counseling hadn't gotten to square one with him. He was resistant, he refused to be open, and he wasn't willing to even identify his problems, much less work on them. Against his will, he was signed into a month-long residential adolescent treatment program, oddly enough at P.I.R., where I'd been hospitalized a few years before. After his evaluation, the team leader sat us down to talk about the issues. Not surprisingly, Gregg was diagnosed with dual problems: depression and alcohol abuse. Yes, the anger was a sign of repressed depression. No, he was not yet an alcoholic, but if he continued on the same path that would in all likelihood become part of his psychology. His autobiography, a required component of intake, was one of the most insightful they'd ever read, but if Gregg "stonewalled" and refused to cooperate, they wouldn't be able to help him. Still, they were skilled with young people, Gregg was intelligent, and they'd do their best to get through his passive-aggressive armor.

As usual, for whatever reason, I was optimistic. I knew the program was exceptional, from my own teaching experience with troubled adolescents, so I expected that this setting, apart from parents and stepparents and siblings and rivals, would address what was going on inside him. Maybe, like me, he'd have a breakthrough. Then he could build from there and continue with therapy and school.

Will paid half of Gregg's private school tuition. He refused to send him back for his junior and senior years to the same boys' school. This created an economic impasse; I couldn't pay the full ride, Will wouldn't pay half. Together we hired an educational consultant, to help us break the stalemate but most particularly to find a place suitable for Gregg. She reviewed his school records, his psychological reports, had separate interviews with Gregg, me and John, Will and Betti, and came up with a recommendation. This boarding school in Maine, The Hyde School, had a wonderful reputation for dealing with troubled boys. Of course, there were the wilderness programs, but Gregg had an intellectual component that needed to be challenged. This particular school was nationally known for its successes with bright boys who had somehow failed in the mainstream. They didn't usually take rising juniors, but she'd called and talked with the admissions officers. She would start the ball rolling for us, if that's what we wanted. We all researched the school and saw it as an excellent option for a fresh start with a sharp focus on Gregg's therapeutic needs. It involved a huge parental time commitment, requiring that parents come periodically for family counseling sessions, plus an almost doubled tuition, but we were ready to do whatever was required to get Gregg healthy again.

John and I visited Gregg regularly at the hospital; so did his dad and that family. We tried to schedule so we wouldn't all be there at the same time. Less tension for Gregg, less tension for all of us. We'd sit outside on the grounds and talk at the picnic tables. Gregg was cryptic, but he'd talk some. He told us he was "furious" that he'd been placed there. He didn't want to go to a school in Maine for his last two years; he wanted to return to his old school. He wasn't responsive to the sessions, wouldn't agree to stop drinking completely, and seemed to be "biding his time" more than making an effort to deal with whatever was making him so angry, uncooperative, and unpredictable. Once a week the teenagers had "group" therapy with the parents. At first, all four of us came; then John refused to go back anymore, saying he hated seeing Gregg like that, plus he thought Will and Betti had more of an agenda to undermine/blame me than to try to get Gregg to be open and honest. The tension in the room felt counterproductive to me, too, I must admit. But I kept going.

The day Gregg was released, on Antabuse so he couldn't drink, we set out for Maine. He had an interview with the admissions officer the next day. A school friend drove since John was tied up with adult classes. Lara's parents gave her permission to come with us, with me chaperoning. Gregg and I talked a lot about "what next?" during this thirteen-hour drive.

"Don't sugarcoat anything during the interview," I cautioned. The school only took students who were willing to be honest about their thoughts, feelings, and experiences. The educational consultant advised that parents, too, had to be open to digging down deep. I hammered the point to Gregg that he should not try to hide behind any defenses, that he should "lay it all out" and answer every question with the unblemished truth. From the educational specialist, I understood that to be essential to acceptance. Will would meet us there, and the three of us would go into the interview together. We'd been warned that this could take hours. We wouldn't be able to hide the friction, so we shouldn't even try.

We stayed with friends that night before the interview. Gregg and Lara fit into the adult group comfortably. We laughed and ate lobsters and talked into the night. As I went to bed I thought, *The hospital helped, despite Gregg's stubbornness; he's at a turning point. Getting him away to a school like this is the right next step, no matter how much it costs.* I actually slept.

I was impressed as we took the tour the next morning. The campus was beautiful—sort of a mini UVA—and the program encouraged respect, self-respect, and responsibility. Away from home and family tensions, Gregg could start over and grow into his "best" self, a self we hadn't seen in months. If anger really had been building up inside him since pre-school, he could work with people who knew how to deal with that. As we walked around, he was polite and guarded, not antagonistic at all.

But apparently, the school's notion of truth and my idea of openness were two different things. In the admissions office, we settled in to be open and honest. Gregg did not sugarcoat; he answered questions like "Why do you want to be here?" with cautious responses. "I'm not sure I do want to be here. My parents think I need help. I guess I do, but I've only been here for a few hours." Will and I were honest, too, Will telling about his frustration with my "humanistic" parenting, me providing my take on how Will and Betti's constant criticism wore away at Gregg's confidence, which he buried deep down, often with alcohol. After four hours of grilling by this attractive, piercing school rep, in which Gregg and Will and I laid ourselves bare, the admissions officer determined that Gregg was too hostile for them to handle. Some kids needed to "hit the bricks" before they were ready for help, the admissions officer announced, and "Gregg is no doubt one of them." I was stunned. They had all his records before our arrival. Who could they have been expecting? Who were the troubled boys they served? Why had we bothered to come, to get our hopes up?

This was an unexpected blow to all three of us, but it was especially a letdown for Gregg. He hadn't been accepted? This had never happened in his life, not ever, and I think he hadn't even considered that as a possibility. Whatever "fresh start" he'd reconciled himself to, even with reluctance, wasn't going to happen. He had been accepted at the Catholic boys' military school Jaison attended, his dad approved of this placement, so he had a "fallback" option. But I thought it was a horrible fit, an invitation to failure at best, some sort of disaster and expulsion at the worst outside possibility. In the first place, his happy-go-lucky brother was a popular rising senior there; Gregg in no way had a shred of Jaison's affable personality. Also, he'd be in Richmond, where he already had a "bad boy" rep. No matter that Richmond's a big city; in prep school circles it's gossip small. But most of all, he didn't want to go, to wear a uniform and march around like a young pretend soldier, but now he wasn't going to have any other options. It was the middle of August; school was going to start the next week. All we were left with was a bad choice.

Gregg and Lara were to ride back to Virginia with Will. I rode home with my friend driving, more bewildered and hopeless than I'd felt in some time. Flabbergasted, in fact.

"Why in the world did she send us up here if they can't work with kids like Gregg?" I asked over and over. "Would we be grabbing at forty-thousand dollar straws if his problems were minor, if he already behaved the way he's supposed to behave, had confidence enough to resist high school temptations?"

That weekend goes down in my mind as a low point. When I finally got home, exhausted, I had a phone call from Gregg. He was crying. Gregg. Crying. He always kept his emotions in check (except for those angry events that stand out like flashing red lights). Betti had called him into a room when his dad was gone and insisted he sit down and hear her out. In front of his younger stepbrother, who Gregg loved, she went on a rant about what a horrible person he was. To her mind, Gregg had deliberately sabotaged the interview at the Maine school just to hurt his dad. He was doing all these bad things with malicious intent to ruin his dad's life and marriage, and it was working. He was going to cause Will to have a heart attack if he kept up his bad behavior. If that happened, Gregg would be the cause of his own daddy's death. Betti wanted Gregg to know in no uncertain terms that she didn't intend to stand by and watch this happen. He needed to know she was onto him.

Gregg, shocked, still reeling from his rejection at the school, begged to come home. I said of course; John would come for him. This was not a habit; for years we'd never intervened on one another's visitation, unless we got the okay ahead of time. But this was cruel, this was kicking Gregg when he was down, and he didn't have to put up with it. Here he was, a seventeen-year-old boy crying because he'd been sucker-punched by this woman who supposedly had his best interests at heart. He hadn't cried once since that sixth-grade fiasco with the school play. This was the guy who had almost never showed his feelings, hadn't even cried much when he was a baby. Betti might call it "crying to Mama"; I called it getting out from a poisonous situation, escaping while the getting away was good. I'd seen first hand how she could attack.

Jaison and I went with Gregg for his interview with the priest who ran the Catholic military school. He talked to Gregg straight on, explaining that he would enter the school with a clean slate. But it would be up to Gregg to keep the slate clean.

"Respect me, respect the rules, you'll get along fine." As a military school, they had two levels of rules, the educational/administrative guidelines and the military mandates. He would have to toe the mark in both realms. I have to admit I liked the way the Father talked directly and frankly to Gregg. He was no-nonsense, yes, but he struck me as fair and intelligent, too. While Jaison hadn't set the world on fire academically while he was there, he'd thrived in his socio-emotional skills. He was well-liked by students and faculty alike, and headed for college with oodles of confidence. Maybe Gregg would land on his feet after all. While I had my doubts about his ability to march to the military drum, others had done it, even easy-going Jaison. Maybe this would be a good choice after all.

He played football that fall. One bizarre incident sticks out in my mind. The football program was lousy. The school had admitted a number of boys for their sports prowess instead of their brains, but it hadn't done any good. They couldn't get a head coach to stay. After one away game, Gregg apparently got into a shouting match on the bus with one of the "stars" who was willing to blame someone else for lost touchdowns. Gregg wasn't taking it, though the jocks were after some weaker guys, not him. It wasn't about him, but he spoke up, and apparently some "we'll settle this later" words were exchanged. The coach was in the front of the bus, clueless, uninvolved with the heckling and threats. When John and I went to meet the bus, the coach told us Gregg had "run off," just disappeared. That made no sense, of course. The coach said he'd gone looking for Gregg, that everyone else had showered and left, that he had no idea why Gregg had "run off." When we found Gregg, still in his uniform lurking behind a tree, he refused to tell us why he'd run away. This was not at all like him. Sometime later he told us he was avoiding a fight, but he didn't tell us what had happened on the bus that night. At the time his erratic behavior was disturbing to us and the school.

Despite a bad football season, Gregg was excited about basketball. The coach at the school was famous in Catholic school circles. When Will and I had first moved to Richmond together, when Melanie was an infant, Will had coached with this man and had the highest respect for both his coaching prowess and his integrity. He knew him well. I was so excited for Gregg to get the opportunity to work with him. He was a disciplinarian, yet he was smart. He ran the team with a strategic eye and a big heart. Everyone who knew him admired him. Plus he was noted for his small, smart point guards. This was a chance for Gregg to get exactly what he needed in the sports arena that he loved so well. He made it to the last round of cuts and didn't make the team. Sports had always been his golden ticket. I don't know when he'd had the wind knocked out of him like that; even the rejection at the school in Maine hadn't hit him like this. Too late, Will called his friend to ask him to reconsider. I have no idea why he didn't call him before the final cuts and talk to him about all of Gregg's great potential as a human being and an athlete, his struggles, his need for this one successful outlet. But the coach had made up his mind; as much talent as Gregg had, he was afraid to take him on because he might cause trouble. Of course, he knew about the weirdo football event. Since Gregg was a junior, why take him on? There would be no clean slate, no second chance. I see this clearly as the moment Gregg gave up and we lost him.

From there on, he went down the tubes academically and socially. In his mind, there was no reward for trying. Yes, he brought a lot of "bad boy" baggage, but he'd never given less than 100% in sports. This was the one thing he wanted at this new school, needed, to hold his head up, and it was squelched. Was this a needed logical consequence, a wake-up call he would heed? He stopped arriving at school on time. He took demerits and wouldn't walk the penalty tours. His shoes and uniform were dirty, and he wouldn't shine or iron anymore, no matter who insisted. The adult in charge of the military, I think he was called the commandant, made threats and Gregg ignored him. He turned in enough work to pass his classes, but just barely. Instead of hanging out with the athletes at school, he started hanging out with the druggies. I'm sure of this; I found out in the worst possible way.

One Friday evening we had friends over. Ours was the household that always had people over, since we had a toddler and a teenager under house arrest. This couple was from out of town, so they'd be spending the night. Gregg was mostly up in his room with his music; when the doorbell rang, I answered. It was Gregg's friend Jordy. He asked if he could tell Gregg hi. Like a fool, I said sure and called Gregg down. They hugged, as our boys do with their friends, and stood talking for a couple of minutes before Jordy left. I stood right there with them the whole time. Gregg went back to his room. I thought, *How nice.*

In the middle of the night, I heard a scream from one of the bedrooms, a blood-chilling scream like I'd never heard in my life. Truly, it sounded like someone was dying. I sat up in bed, terrified. Something was grievously wrong. John jumped up, told me to stay put. When I tried to follow him, he insisted I stay in the bedroom. By now our friend was up, too. The screaming went on, and I heard John and Tom go into Gregg's bedroom across the hall. I literally held my breath. What had happened?

John came back, took my hands, and sat me down. "Gregg's on a bad acid trip." ACID? Where did Gregg get Acid??? "Tom and I will stay with him. He'll be all right, but it'll take time. You cannot, under any circumstances, get up. You can't see him." And I didn't. Miranda was still asleep. The men would know what to do. By morning, he'd be all right.

I prayed and cried and sat up. By morning, John and Tom told me Gregg was "down" and all right. He'd be sleeping for a while.

"What happened? How did this happen?" At this point I was numb; my logical brain hadn't figured it out.

"Jordy brought him blotter acid last night. Gregg took a lot, too much."

"Acid? He could've died?"

"Yeah, but he's okay now." John hugged me. He and Tom had lived a different sixties, in large universities. I'd gone to Mary Washington. I'd never even seen pot, much less acid, in college. Thank God they'd known what to do.

Ironically, Jordy lived with his dad. "I'm going to call Jordy's father." I usually avoid confrontation, but this time I didn't hesitate; I called. I told him if he didn't deal with Jordy I'd call the police. He promised he would. Who knows? I didn't tell the school. Perhaps that was irresponsible, but John and I decided not to. We wanted Gregg to graduate. We'd be certain not to let any more of his buddies near him after school hours. During the day, the school would be in loco parentis, and they were already watching Gregg closely.

Will wanted to have more involvement with Gregg and that suited me to a T. Since Gregg had always been an exceptional baseball player, Will got his college roommate, also a VMI grad and a college baseball coach, to sponsor a Scratoma league team with him. These were guys too old for Little League any longer. Gregg agreed to play. Again, I was optimistic. Will's roommate, Denny, was Gregg's Godfather. He'd known Gregg, though peripherally, since he was born. He knew about his problems from A to Z. Both Will and Denny were "tough love" kinds of coaches, but perhaps that's what Gregg needed. That's what they believed, anyway, and who was I to fault them? I wasn't getting anywhere.

At the beginning, Gregg's complaints were legit. I'd go to the games, at first. They'd get up in his face and yell at him. He'd take it. They'd sit him on the bench. He'd take it. They'd criticize every little thing, never say "great job" when he got a base hit or made a good fielding play. He'd take it. Was he just being a jerk, or was he a victim? I have no way of knowing.

Eventually, he started deliberately slacking. This sent both Will and Denny into fits, but he ignored them. In the end, they had to kick him off the team, and he deserved it. For whatever reason, tough love didn't work. Maybe it was the double-teaming, maybe he was playing poor pitiful Gregg, or maybe it was too late. Sports were over for him.

That summer, John and I needed some R & R. Gregg had been grounded the last half of his junior year. He'd been kicked off the recreational baseball team. If we couldn't get him to be responsible and to make somewhat sensible decisions, we could at least keep him at home under our watch, but that had been draining, too. He no longer went to his father's on weekends, so we were constantly "on duty." One weekend in late summer, when Melanie and Gregg were both home and Jaison was with his mother, John and I decided to go to Lexington to see some friends. We'd take Miranda with us. Melanie had a waitressing job for the summer; she'd be in charge of the house, but not of Gregg. He'd eat and sleep there, but their paths shouldn't cross too much. Since his problems, she'd steered clear of him, and that suited Gregg fine. He was working construction, making spending money for college. John worried about leaving those two in the house, but I had to get away.

As usual, John was right. In the middle of Saturday night, we got a frantic call from Melanie. She was furious and scared. Gregg was having a party. She'd gone downstairs to beg him to please keep it down or neighbors would probably call the police. He'd gotten furious with her; she felt threatened. They'd cursed one another, and now she was upstairs on the third floor locked in her room. We needed to come home right away, because even right away meant two and a half more hours. We assured her we would, got Miranda up, put her to sleep in the back seat, and headed home to Richmond, John angry enough to spit nails, me worried sick.

100

When we got there the house was a wreck—even a lacy bra in the hallway to the kitchen, such a cliché— and Gregg was gone. Melanie was furious with us for leaving her with him. School opening couldn't arrive soon enough to suit me.

After every one of these previous fiascos, Gregg and I had talked long and hard about learning from his mistakes, about what he needed to do to get his head on straight, about how people perceived him and what he wanted from life. We always talked. Up to this point, he and I could talk openly. Or maybe I talked and kidded myself that he was listening. This time I had nothing to say. I let John talk. Perhaps talk is too polite a word. John told him off in no uncertain terms. He'd disrespected us, he'd disrespected our home, he'd frightened his sister; what the hell was wrong with him? He'd need to clean the place up, he'd need to talk to his buddies who'd taken some of our belongings and get them to bring them back, he'd need to repair the broken chair—and not sometime in the future, now. John and Gregg had always gotten along well, but this was a breaking point. Gregg did what he was told, he was cowed, but he had trashed our home and crossed a line with John, and he knew it.

That spring had been strange in more ways than just Gregg's problems. Jaison would take Miranda for walks around the block; often she'd ride her Big Wheel. One early evening, Jaison came home laughing about an absurd incident. This guy, obviously "not right," was hiding in the bushes, creeping along behind them. It was almost like a grown man playing hide and seek, he told us. We lived in an old neighborhood with grand old homes—the governor lived half a block down the street—but we also had a "haunted house" on our block and low-rent apartments only a few streets away. It was "Southern Gothic" in a good way, or so we'd thought. A few afternoons later, Jaison didn't laugh after the two of them had taken their walk. The same man had followed them again, only this time he'd spoken to Jaison.

"Hey, you, is that your little sister?" Jaison glared at him. "Well if it is, you'd better watch her. Ain't safe to have a pretty little girl out on the streets." This gave us all the creeps.

I'd grown up in Richmond. Years before, I'd gone to high school with a guy who'd become an undercover detective. We called him and described what had happened. Jaison gave me and John a full description of the guy. The next evening, when he was off duty, my classmate came over, sat on our front porch, and off the record, told us who the man was and showed us his rap sheet. He was living in a halfway house nearby. He had a string of sexual offenses as long as my arm. The latest involved exposing himself to a room full of women exercising during lunch hour in a professional building downtown. We had Jaison repeat what he'd said, word for word. Johnny X. told us we could file a complaint, but the police wouldn't be able to do a thing. He hadn't threatened Jaison or Miranda; his words wouldn't "meet the legal standard." But he himself would be glad to pick the creep up on his motorcycle, drag him into one of the dark alleys in our neighborhood, break his legs, and tell him to stay away from our block. That was all he could do for us until he actually threatened my children. We couldn't take him up on his offer. A few weeks later, the guy was arrested for "touching" two sisters at a nearby playground. Miranda began to have "bad thoughts," fearful of being out of our sight for too long, even during the school day.

That May, I had finished my M.F.A. in creative writing. For my thesis, I'd written a first draft of a novel. I could go back to teaching in the prep school where I'd previously worked, or I could look for a college position. The academic landscape was barren where we lived, with no full-time academic positions open in the area. Melanie was graduating from college; she would be moving to New Orleans, finding an apartment and a legal job there. Jaison was leaving for college. We wouldn't need all that space anymore. John and I had talked about moving; perhaps the time was right to get away, to put some distance between me and my hometown. We looked toward the western part of the state, where the cost of living was considerably less expensive. Perhaps I could work part-time as an adjunct and write. The hitch was that Gregg had one more year of high school. How would he fare in a huge consolidated rural high school, especially as a senior? John was willing to stay behind with him. He'd get a modest two-bedroom apartment; perhaps he and Gregg, by themselves, in a less stressful setting, could make things work.

We found a small home in the mountains. I got a job teaching two nights a week in a nearby community college. Miranda would have to ride the school bus, but that didn't strike me as much of a problem. Lots of children rode the school bus. John could come home on Fridays; Gregg could come with him or go to his dad's.

Miranda and I did fine, but John and Gregg both had a dreadful nine months. Gregg started off cooperating, but that tapered off, until he eventually disappeared on weekends. He wasn't hanging with the jocks, so the likelihood was that he was back in with his drug buddies. John could either stay and search for him or come home and worry. In any case, we'd worry, so he'd come home.

Gregg did graduate, but he was told he could not attend the commencement exercises. That was fair. He had so many demerits by then they had to do something. We had a sad little celebration dinner on my mother's deck. Gregg didn't feel attached to that school and he didn't act as if he cared about being "uninvited" to his own graduation Actually, he smiled and talked more that night than he had in some time. He'd never play organized sports again. He'd lost so much in such a short time, but he'd managed to hold onto his intelligence and learn, despite his bad behaviors. He'd done well enough academically to gain acceptance at a competitive Virginia university. In late August, he'd be in an adult environment making his own decisions. We'd done the best we could. Thank God he'd graduated, even if it was under a cloud.

Strangely, he had been accepted at James Madison University for the fall. That had been contingent on his successful completion of high school, so we had been holding our breath and hoping he'd keep it together at least enough to get to college. So we all did feel a sense of relief, if not happiness, at that gathering. In college, it would be up to him. The evening was more celebratory than we'd expected.

Gregg tried working construction that summer for his father, but the project supervisor had to fire him for insolence. It didn't appear that he was learning from his mistakes after all. As far as we were all concerned, he couldn't get away to college fast enough.

Before school got underway, Gregg had one more brush with the law, a bad one. The graduated seniors had apparently planned one big end of summer blow-out before they all went their separate ways. I'd gone back home. Gregg was working, doing pickup construction, staying with his dad or his buddies. After work, he went wherever he wanted to go. I couldn't hand-hold any more, and hand holding hadn't done a bit of good anyway. What difference did it make? I admit I had no control over him, but neither had school or his dad. I have no idea if Gregg was invited to this party or not; I tend to think he crashed. In any case, he and two buddies went late, after things were well under way. Gregg was drunk, driving, swerving in front of the house. Many of the teenagers were out front. Apparently he almost ran down one of the girls, a younger daughter of one of my good friends, Miranda's former nanny. Later that night, Gregg and the guys he was with went back and vandalized the two side-by-side homes where the party had been held. I didn't know about any of this at the time, not until he was arrested.

I went to court with him but would not speak for him. These days he was insisting that his behavior was "overblown," that he'd never ever intended to hit a friend with the car, that he didn't participate in the damage. Excuses, excuses, excuses, no taking ownership for his actions. Scary. As a parent, it was my obligation to be there; as a human being, I in no way condoned or excused what he had done. He and the two other boys were assigned community service, payment of all repair costs, and payment of court costs. When they completed their punishment, their records would be expunged if they'd kept their noses clean. This was serious, and costly. Far worse than wrecking our car. This was a side of Gregg, a bitter drinking side, that was nothing but bad news. I could only hope that the judgment of the court would shake him up in ways I'd never been able to.

John and I drove with him to college in August, both cars packed with his belongings. Gregg was actually excited; a fresh start away from his hometown and siblings and parents made him optimistic. His dorm, even clean, looked like the run-down victim of constant partying. No white columns and parlors with grand pianos here. This double room of his was institutional décor at its barest. We sat on his unmade bed in this dreary, uninviting room. Our talk was as solemn and somber as I felt.

"Gregg, this is it, Boog. You've got what you want; you're gonna be on your own."

"I know that, Mom."

"So don't blow it."

"I don't want to."

"I love you, you know that."

"I love you."

"So be smart. Be safe. Do what's right." We stood and hugged. "Use that big brain of yours for a change." I was near tears. I left so John could go in and have his talk.

I don't know what they said, but they came out arm in arm. Gregg and I hugged again, and then we waved goodbye and walked to our car. John and I didn't talk much on the way home. We both wanted this to work. I know John was thinking Gregg didn't have a chance. I didn't want to think that too, but at this point it was hard to be upbeat, even for me.

CHAPTER 7 -- COMMITMENT

Our family was undergoing major changes. Miranda and I had spent a lot of time by ourselves in our remote rural home during Gregg's senior year in military school while he and John shared an apartment in Richmond. We loved Miranda's second grade teacher, Ms. Marie Coleman; she was funny and encouraging and found Miranda delightful, so Miranda had a positive year, making lots of school friends. As a "baby" in a huge family for the first seven years of her life, she'd moved, now, to an "only" in an isolated mountain family of three—two most days of the week. Ms. Coleman loved singing and making art and drama, just like Miranda, so she felt happy in her boisterous classroom. At the year's end, Ms. Coleman gave Miranda a special gift—plastic garlic earrings, to ward off any "evil spirits." Her "bad thoughts" stopped.

Few children lived nearby, though. Miranda was the first child on the rural bus in the morning and the last off in the evening. While she didn't really like the hour-plus bus ride, she didn't complain much about it. Next on after her was a boy neighbor from down the road who already hunted at eight years old. Miranda liked him all right, but the two didn't have much in common. They couldn't be characterized as friends, but they got along.

That first year, John came to our new mountain home on weekends, but he'd be so stressed about Gregg that he was often tense and grumpy. The second year he would be with us full-time—well, mostly full-time. He'd stay over in Richmond from Tuesday through Thursday, with a dear friend, teaching adult classes part-time in the evening. With my adjunct teaching, we'd be okay financially, but just barely. Jaison and Gregg were both in college. They liked coming to the mountains on occasion, but weren't with us often. On two part-time salaries, we couldn't afford to travel to New Orleans to visit Melanie. She only came home at Christmas, so we saw her in Richmond at my mother's. Except for me, John, and Miranda, our family was suddenly scattered.

I'd teach when and where I could, summer school included. I was finishing my second novel, a first-person story of a young woman examining her marriage in the context of her husband's sports career. A different small press had it under contract, and I was overjoyed when I sent in the first draft. That thrill didn't last long. The editor/owner had praised the book, and we were set to work together on revisions. Somewhere in the process she'd hired an assistant, an artist/writer with an ego way more refined than his manners. The letter he sent regarding the re-write was rude to the point of insulting—along the "read Fitzgerald before your next draft" lines. I wrote back saying it was clear to me that we wouldn't be able to work together. My failure to submit the rewrite in six months would in essence nullify the contract. It was a painful letter to write. I submitted that novel to another small press and received a lovely rejection (Is that an oxymoron?). The literary editors accepted the manuscript; the marketing editors said they couldn't sell it. I put the manuscript in a drawer and indulged in some rather weepy sessions. John, as an artist himself, kept reminding me that "making art is about the process, not about publishing," but I couldn't help longing for acceptance and validation through my writing. What should've been a happy time for us, with our move and three of the four children "launched," was in truth pretty gloomy.

Lucky coincidence, John returned from Richmond one weekend with a call for novel manuscripts from Style magazine no bigger than a want ad. "Small start-up publisher seeks literary novels…"

He confessed "I really like your thesis novel better than this one," and I felt a little bit superstitious about the bad karma already attached to the second book, so I decided to submit the first instead. What could I lose? The novel was accepted, and I was on my feet again, in terms of a sense that I could have a writing life as well as a teaching career.

And Gregg surprised us his first semester in college; he did fine, academically. He didn't come home much—our mountain place had never really been his home, as he reminded us often. He'd made some friends, his grades were a bit above average, and he hadn't gotten into any trouble we knew about. This was a definite improvement, an upswing.

His second semester grades were awful; he failed a few classes, got C's and D's in others. He would return in the fall on academic probation, but at least he could return. At that point we were thankful for small blessings, even teensy ones. He decided he wanted to work at Nags Head for the summer, so he got permission from my parents to stay in the "bunkhouse" in one of their cottages. Jaison was headed to Alaska to work on a salmon fishing boat for the twelve weeks between semesters. Melanie was still in New Orleans, working as a paralegal. This all felt normal, since our ongoing worries about Gregg were standard operating procedure, and at least at this moment they were school-related, not mental-health related.

John and I met other couples with children Miranda's age in our community, really through her schoolmates, and we'd get together for cookouts and potlucks that summer. Overall life was slower, less stressed. I joined a writers' group. Some of our new friends were musicians, artists, and writers. Evenings we'd build bonfires and have impromptu old-time music outdoors. I supplemented our income by writing for the local weekly. Country living was different, but to all outward appearances our lives settled and all three of us felt happier. I started going to a nearby Quaker Meeting and Miranda went with me. Gregg called occasionally; he wasn't making much money, but he was learning to surf and sounded happy.

Miranda's second year in her rural school, in third grade, she had a "drill sergeant" of a teacher. She began to complain about the bus ride, the little boy at her table who stuck out his tongue at her and teased her while the teacher's back was turned, and the "mean" teacher herself. We began to get calls during the day. Miranda was sick; she was crying, had put her head down, and wouldn't do her work. At home her "bad thoughts" returned, and she began calling in to us every night, "Are you alright, Mom? Say you're alright." Our attention diverted from Gregg, who seemed to be settling into college, albeit on probation, to her. I wasn't about to let any red flags regarding her emotional health flap in my face without doing something right away.

We took her to a clinical social worker at the local mental health center. At her advice, the three of us went into family counseling. We began to work on the underlying stress and tension in our home. John didn't like the weekly traveling back and forth to Richmond. When he came home, I expected not only help with Miranda and the household responsibilities, but personal attention as well. In truth, I was starved for John's attention. While I had plenty of "Charlotte" time during the week, Charlotte + John time was a thing of the past. We weren't having a couple of beers on the deck together after Miranda's bedtime; he wasn't able to laugh about the small stories Miranda and I hoarded for him—he needed to vent about the year before with Gregg, how awful it had been for him. From his perspective, he expected some understanding, some affection, and some much-needed time to himself. He'd purchased the old post office in the town nearby and spent considerable weekend time there renovating it as his studio. Between traveling, teaching, and working on his studio, he wasn't getting to make art, which always made him irritable. Neither of us was getting our needs met, and each tended to blame it on the other. That's easy to do "long distance." Miranda was feeling pretty alone and lonely, fifteen miles out of the closest town, no doubt sensing the tension between her parents as well. The evening babysitter I'd hired, who came with her daughter who was Miranda's age while I taught two night classes, was hands-off to the point of being negligent. As a family we had to make some changes; this had nothing to do with Gregg.

Meanwhile, Gregg had decided that instead of a dorm he would live in a house with some of his buddies that sophomore fall. We had taken our contribution of second-hand furniture to his place and checked it out. While I wasn't big on this change, I had to admit that the house was more welcoming than the dorm. He wanted to be in college, so we told ourselves he'd do whatever it took to get by, to make his grades. He always had been brain smart, even if his judgment was skewed. But first semester he got in trouble pulling fire alarms in a dorm, and since he was on probation he got kicked out for the rest of the year. This was disturbing, of course, and disruptive to our already stressed family situation. What was even more disturbing was Gregg's refusal to take any responsibility for his behavior. He insisted that "other guys did the same thing all the time," and he was "taking the rap." We strived to get the severity of what he'd done across to him.

"No matter what other people do, you're in charge of YOU. What you did was dead wrong. You endangered the safety of the entire dorm." His attitude was lackadaisical, inappropriate; his reasoning was childlike at best, irrational at worst. In his mind, it "wasn't a big deal," and the consequences in no way fit the crime. He wanted to stay put in the college town, to work and get back into school as soon as possible. Since this was a logical plan, we didn't argue. He'd wait tables and re-apply when his suspension was up.

That didn't work either. He got fired from the waiting job and began to be a job gypsy, from pizza delivery to dishwashing to sweeping floors. One of his housemates "had it in for him." He'd never liked that guy anyway. Every time we talked, he was in some kind of minor trouble. Finally, he came to stay with us. Since we only had two bedrooms, he'd "fix up" the work building we had out back by the creek. It had electricity and a poured concrete floor, but no heat except for a small wood stove. We heated with wood ourselves, so we didn't see that as particularly "roughing it." Jaison was doing well in school. Melanie was in New Orleans, engaged to her college sweetheart. John and Miranda and I continued our counseling. Gregg needed to go to work and get his act together.

One weekend when the three of us were away and Gregg was "housesitting" for us and feeding our animals, John came home early to find him in the living room with a group of his buddies, a keg of beer, drug paraphernalia, and a tank of hydrogen, the kind used to blow up party balloons. They were all high as kites. John kicked the guys out and sent Gregg to his "cabin."

John knew the deal: people used the hydrogen in combination with the pot for some sort of super-high. He told me later that all night long cars continued to drive up into our driveway and he had to tell guys the party was off. The next day, we had a serious talk with Gregg.

We told him, in no uncertain terms, "You can't live with us if you're going to bring drugs and characters we don't know into the house; we have Miranda to consider. Do you actually think this is okay, in our home, with your little sister?" And "You know this could lead to legal problems and put our jobs and even our safety in jeopardy." He wasn't supposed to be using drugs in the first place. If he wanted to stay, he'd have to sign a contract promising no more drugs, no more parties, and no drinking and driving.

For once, Gregg was actually remorseful. He apologized—John and I both took it as sincere, and John's no easy sell—and we took him at his word. He swore he wanted to stay with us and stay clean. He signed the contract. John was skeptical, I was hopeful: mini breakthrough, Gregg apologizing?

I was working at the local community college and newspaper. John was working part-time teaching studio art in Richmond. He'd come home and we'd go to our therapist on Friday afternoons after Miranda got out of school. On hindsight, that wasn't much of a howdy-do for us as a couple each week. We'd hope there would be no new "Gregg situation" that week. Sometimes we'd see friends on Saturday night; sometimes John would work on the studio. He'd leave Sunday afternoon. To say our marriage was floundering would be an understatement; both of us knew we weren't happy, but neither of us was taking a single step, outside the therapy sessions, to address the problems. We grabbed our laughs where we could find them, hoping tensions would ease and we'd find our way back to one another.

One early summer Saturday, we cleared the calendar for just the three of us. That Friday afternoon, John stayed at the studio, and he had a breakthrough of sorts. Drawing, he began to create these large fantastical colorful animals. One looked like some sort of red bull; another, like a giant black crow. For the first time in months he had that creative high going. Miranda had been singing in the little choir at the Baptist church in the town nearby. She had a "recital" of sorts, along with the "graduation" of Vacation Bible School. We would attend that on Saturday afternoon and then go to the county fair. While it sounds like a simple, even boring, evening, it was a stand-out.

John and I are both spiritual but not religious. We wanted Miranda to have a sense of neighborhood, but she was a fish out of water in that little rural community. As she likes to say, her best friend was the seventy-five-year-old woman down the lane. A remarkable woman, but in any case, a peculiar best friend for a nine-year-old. So for two weeks, we'd gone to Vacation Bible School together, Miranda and I, for social interaction more than religious instruction. I'd been a Baptist as a child, before the hypocrisy of the Civil Rights Movement, when I left the church. I'd attended and taught Vacation Bible School myself. So I agreed to teach crafts and go with Miranda, feeling a bit odd but nonetheless pleased for the opportunity to be with her, having fun. We could talk about anything religious that confused her. She had girls her age to play with every morning for a couple of weeks.

The graduation ceremony this particular Saturday turned out to be upbeat and funny. I loved singing the old Baptist hymns, always have. The pianist was a sharp minister's wife who taught English at the community college with me. She could make that stand-up piano shake. Miranda looked so adorable in the choir's front row, with a black lace mantilla she'd chosen for the "special occasion" covering her head. We both dressed in somewhat oddball "outfits" at that time, and I loved her sense of the fey. John, in a lighthearted mood, was amused by it all—the whole country Baptist scene struck him as a skit out of *Saturday Night Live*—he'd been raised a Lutheran, and such frivolous celebrations were not part of his church experience. When the rather large woman who supervised VBS stood up to give her thanks to the volunteers, he almost lost it ("Wide-ette," he whispered, nearly cracking up; we connected). I swear I elbowed him to shush. I was called up front and given a Whirl-a-Gig made out of neon plastic popsicle sticks as a sign of the church's gratitude for my service. I almost sat somewhere else afterwards, John was so red in the face.

"What the hell is that thing?" he whispered, stifling an outburst. But he made it through the service, and I didn't care for one second about his irreverence. The fact that the three of us were laughing and having a good time felt more important to me than honoring the Lord's house. Any God worth caring for was laughing, too.

We went to the fair about a half mile down the road from the church, behind the firehall. We ate gross yummy fair food. John and Miranda rode the Tilt-a-Whirl and the Ferris Wheel. Again, we were having a blast together.

John pointed. "Would you look at that?" At one concession stand, a baby about two was sitting on the edge of the counter drinking Coca-Cola from his bottle. The tendrils of our wry shared sense of humor connected us, and we had to laugh. A group of teenagers was running through the crowd pushing a newborn in an Umbrolla; the baby's head rocked from side to side. He couldn't have been more than six weeks old, his head bobbling like a bobble doll. His scrawny, red-headed mama, clad in a denim mini-skirt and bustier, smoking, sauntered along behind the kids on her platform heels. More than once we all wished we were photographers so we could've captured this "tilted world." Driving through the mountains toward home, the sun setting, all three of us declared that this was the most fun we'd had in forever.

We heard the phone ringing as we walked up the front steps. John and I were laughing about where to hang the Whirl-a-Gig on the porch. I remember that distinctly, that final sunset glow, us laughing in the clear evening air. It was John's nephew Marc calling. I watched as, silent, John's face melted from silly to somber. John's dad was dead; he'd died that day of a heart attack, his first. John was devastated. He was a late-in-life child, the only natural son of both his father and mother. This was a shock; with all the family tension going on, we hadn't seen John's parents that Christmas, for the first time in years.

John kept saying, "Dad's dead; Marc told me he just said 'I'm going, Mary,' and he died, right there in the living room with Mom, sitting up in his chair."

I made John go to bed, and I called to get all the information and make the arrangements for us to leave for upstate New York the next morning.

John insisted, "You don't have to go," but I was adamant: of course I'd be with him and his family for this. Miranda, so super sensitive, would stay in Richmond with my parents and Melanie, who'd trade off taking care of her. We'd be gone as long as we needed to be gone.

Gregg was working construction as a helper during this period. We hardly saw him; he hung out with friends down by the river more than he stayed in his place. We didn't make any pretense of supervising him. He claimed to be saving money to go back to school. John was certain he was drinking away his paychecks. In any case, we left the house and animals in his care and took off the next morning. I drove the whole way. John could hardly open his eyes.

His mother was helpless in the face of Jack's death. Everyone had thought she'd "go first," she had so many health problems. John's two older brothers (biological half brothers who'd been adopted by his dad as children) pretty much took over, which was a blessing. The service was moving. Jack had been a mainstay of his small community, and all the civic organizations he'd supported sent representatives who spoke about his contributions. When we got back to the house after the reception at the church, while we were gathering at home in that quiet after-it's-all-over family sad calm, I got a phone call. I panicked. Something was wrong with Miranda! It was Gregg, though. He was in jail in Henrico County. He'd been picked up in our county for some traffic offense. While he was in jail there, they found out he'd broken his earlier parole by not completing some aspect of his community service, and he would await trial until someone posted bail. He expected me to come right away, that day. His dad wouldn't post bail. I surprised myself and Gregg by telling him that John needed me, I wanted to be with his family right then, and he'd have to stay put until I could get there, which would be at least another day or two. He slammed the phone down, furious. I called neighbors to feed our animals. I hated to tell John what was going on, but I had to. Even in the face of his dad's unexpected death, John and I were forced to deal with Gregg's relentless problems.

That night was a low point in our marriage. Because so many relatives were in from out of town for the funeral, John and I were sleeping at a neighbor's home two doors down from Jack and Mary's. John went out drinking with his nephew Marc—I couldn't blame him—but he never came to bed with me that night. I was crushed and scared and totally by myself. No matter what, we always slept together.

Small talk with our hosts was more than I could manage, so I went up to bed early. My son was in jail, my husband didn't want to be with me. I knew who he was with—that wasn't the issue—but I also knew he didn't want me there with him any longer. Alone, lonely: those words are too small to explain the huge emptiness and fear I felt as I lay awake, waiting, all that night.

The next day, exhausted and at my wit's end, I drove back from upstate New York to Richmond alone. I went to my parents' house, and Melanie and I went to the jail to bail out Gregg. Seeing him in handcuffs and shackles, looking at me with near-hatred in his eyes, I hit bottom. Melanie, who was about to enter law school at the time, was furious with him. He no sooner signed the release papers than he lit into us.

"Why didn't you come sooner?" he glared. "Melanie, why the hell didn't you come alone, since Mom was in New York with John? What kind of sister are you?" Everyone else was to blame; he was still the victim. They screamed at one another all the way back to my mother's. I was on the verge of tears. I begged them to stop. Miranda didn't need to see her brother and sister fighting like rabid dogs. They stopped, but Melanie became estranged from Gregg since that day. He never acknowledged his part in their rift, his unreasonable expectation of everyone in the family to rescue him any time he messed up.

Melanie and I turned Gregg over to his father as soon as we could. Instead of heading home, I decided to take Miranda to my parent's beach cottage, the only safe place I thought I could possibly get my head together. My family was in shreds, and I didn't have any solutions. Gregg went back to our place, thinking he would go back to work. He eventually settled his court case; I have no idea how. Neither his dad nor I helped him.

I'm sure he used the excuse that his grandfather had died to cover for his time off. By this time Gregg lied about anything to cover himself. He was already in trouble with this particular boss, though. Two or three of the workers would meet at a pre-determined point every morning and head toward jobsites in close-by big cities. The pay was good. Gregg had been warned about being late. When he wasn't on time, he would hold up an entire crew, and time was money. He hadn't called from jail, so he lost this job, anyway, but again he insisted it wasn't actually his fault. There were plenty of legitimate reasons why he couldn't be there or be on time.

"The boss is a jerk—he didn't like me, anyway. The guy should've given me some slack because Jack died." As always, the boss had been unfair and Gregg deserved limitless chances.

He had a hard time finding work in our rural community, so he decided to head back to Richmond and go to school, to the community college this time. He could get his two-year electronics degree. With that, he could get plenty of work. I let him go with a heartfelt sigh of relief. The nobody-likes-me and my-dad-wants-to-see-me-fail refrains didn't ring true any longer. He refused to own part of the blame when things went wrong, so he was stuck in the same old self-absorbed cycle. With John in shreds and our marriage in jeopardy, we couldn't keep him with us any anyway. I'm not sure he ever even told John he was sorry about Jack's death. By this time, Gregg was in his own world, and though all of the signs were there, I didn't recognize the cause of much of his unrealistic thinking as mental illness. His steady diet of drugs and alcohol masked the deep cause from me.

John and I acknowledged that things had to change between us. We either had to live together full-time and commit to our marriage, or we had to split. We loved each other, without doubt, so we decided to try harder. He got a college teaching job closer to home, a forty-five minute drive each way, but he'd only be working three days a week, so he could do it. I was hired full-time at the community college, only twenty minutes away, and we both believed that despite our long list of troubles we could be happy together, so we re-committed to making things work.

Gregg did get his electricians' degree in two years, with all A's, and his dad helped him get the needed tools and connected him with people in the construction field. Finally, here was a good chance for him to be on his own, making a sufficient income to live independently. With enough hours as an electrician's apprentice, he could get his license. Down the road, he might have his own business. Plenty of bright young men became successful without college degrees. Maybe this was his path. After all, his dad was a civil engineer and had a successful career as part owner/vice president of an enormous company. Perhaps this degree was Gregg's first step toward planting his feet, taking charge of his own life.

He worked with an electrical sub-contractor doing a job on one of Will's large urban renovation projects. He started out poorly. Since he was working on an upper floor, instead of going downstairs to the Port-a-Potty, he decided to urinate in the corner of his work area.

When his supervisor found this out, he of course reprimanded Gregg and warned him, "Any more screw-ups, I'll have to let you go." Probably he didn't can him at that moment because Will was his boss and he had to cut his son a break. This was outrageous behavior on my son's part, but Gregg laughed off my "prudishness." Guys did these things all the time, he claimed.

"The fuckin' boss has it in for me." He wondered what "the big deal" was. Before long, he overslept past his lunch hour and was fired anyway.

Out of work, Gregg went for financial aid and decided to go back to a four-year college. He applied and was accepted at the large urban university in my hometown; his community college degree was a "pass go" to a four-year school. He'd started playing guitar, and he loved it. For a while he had some thought of majoring in music, but when he took the first classes and found out how rigorous the program was and how advanced the other students were, he decided to take lessons and continue to play, but to major in English. At this point in his life, he was handsome and healthy; in external appearance he was fine, even attractive. I was glad he'd found another talent, since he'd given up on sports, and electronics was "just a job." Now that he had a focus and a plan, perhaps he'd settle down. Maybe he'd been through his "druggie/alkie" phase. No doubt he was still way too self-centered, but he'd always been socially delayed. Brain theory suggested males didn't develop frontal brain judgment until the late twenties. A mom could hope. In any case, at this point I was again optimistic that he would turn his life around.

He started off well that first semester, getting solid grades, even taking and loving creative writing, although he claimed that his American Lit. professor, an African-American woman, didn't like him because of his contrary take on Huckleberry Finn. Instead of seeing this as a beginning sign of paranoia, I took it as another example of Gregg's deliberate anti-social, counter-cultural, rebellious behavior. Living alone for once, he adopted a stray kitten. I was pleased, since caring for an animal struck me as a small extension of Gregg beyond his own selfish needs. Soon, though, he claimed that the guy above him had deliberately hurt his pet. Gregg left the screen up so the cat could come and go from his second-floor apartment. One day the kitty came home limping. Gregg was certain, beyond doubt, that the guy upstairs didn't like him or his cat and had thrown it out of the third-floor window. That didn't make a bit of sense to me. In any case, Gregg moved in with some other guys in the same neighborhood. The cat had to go to the SPCA.

Melanie married that Thanksgiving. She was in her third year in law school, and she married another law student. It was a lovely wedding, with the reception at Will's country home. Gregg was not invited; those two had never mended their rift, and I did not intend to alienate either one by imposing any kind of artificial "ought-tos." She didn't want him there, and I respected her choice. It was her wedding.

While Jaison was in town for the wedding, he went to visit Gregg. They'd always been "best friends," had never really had words. This time they got in a fist fight. I never knew the cause, but I think for the first time Jaison understood at a deep level why we were all so concerned about Gregg.

Not many weeks later, Will got an unexpected call from one of Gregg's new roommates. The other two guys asked Will to come over one evening to talk about Gregg, which he did. They claimed Gregg was not pulling his load in terms of the "communal agreement" they'd drawn up, plus he was staying up all hours of the night playing music too loud, as well as taking food that wasn't his from the fridge. They'd tried to talk to him about his responsibilities, but he'd only laughed off their requests. They wanted Will to know—since he'd co-signed for the lease—that they'd give Gregg another month, but if he didn't shape up he'd have to leave. Will talked to Gregg, as he described all this to me, and Gregg was cavalier about it. So he left a few cans around, so he didn't wash a few dishes, so he didn't take out some trash or ate a few bowls of somebody else's cereal. Big deal. So what? Okay, he'd get it straight. Will and I were both concerned about this blatant unwillingness on Gregg's part to maintain his agreement with these guys, but still neither of us realized there was a bigger problem. Both of us viewed Gregg as selfish and inconsiderate at this time in his life. Will was paying for college expenses, as he'd promised, but if Gregg didn't shape up, the gravy train would stop and let him off. This struck me as logical and reasonable.

Christmas holidays intervened. Gregg came up to visit us for a few days. I was pleased to see him; he'd brought his guitar. We talked about recipes and cooking, and for the most part, he seemed to be his best self. But on the last day of his visit, he and John got into a screaming match, getting up in one another's faces and yelling obscenities.

Gregg said horrible things, like, "You sponge off Mom, you always have, you're an asshole," and John was spouting equally cruel remarks: "You're a selfish baby who quits every time it gets tough." I have no idea what started this argument, but I do know it ended with me fearing that John or Gregg or both of them would throw a fist. Gregg had to leave, that was unquestionable. He'd said nasty, hateful things to John. And John had had it. I was in tears as I followed Gregg out to his truck.

"What's wrong with you? Why are you so angry at us—and the world?" He was swearing and rambling on about John never liking him and being mean to me, but he did hug me goodbye. Another sad disaster of a holiday.

Gregg went back to school, and I didn't call him or hear from him for a while. My parents would have him over for dinner on occasion; they'd give him a twenty or take him for a haircut. My mother would call to tell me how sweet Gregg was, and how "cold" we were to keep our distance. Sometimes they'd take him out to eat at their favorite Greek restaurant. I was pleased that they could continue to have a normal relationship with him when he'd alienated most everyone else. At this point, my parents had never experienced bizarro-Gregg.

At the end of February, the roommate called Will again. Gregg would have to go. One of the young men owned a ceremonial sword that he'd hung on the wall in the living room. Gregg was showing an off-the-charts interest in it. They weren't just concerned about house rules any longer, either. They were worried about safety. Will went by to sit down and talk with the two guys. What exactly was Gregg doing? One said that at night, when he was studying, he'd hear Gregg in his room behind closed doors talking. He wasn't talking on the phone, since he didn't have a phone in his room. The other said that no matter the topic, Gregg would babble on about his civil rights, that he'd quote the U.S. Constitution. Gregg had been told to leave the sword alone, but still they'd come home and it would be on the coffee table. Gregg had to go, right away. Will agreed to get a truck that weekend and move him out

Will called me. Would I come to Richmond and meet with him and Gregg? The three of us needed to sit down and try to figure out what was happening. He wouldn't tell Gregg he had to move until we were all together. He didn't want to upset him while he was still living under the same roof with the other two students. That could lead to a blow-up, which we wanted to avoid. I, of course, agreed to come immediately. We decided that first I would call Gregg to see if he'd have lunch with me that Friday. Of course Will would join us, but we knew that that secret "sin of omission" was the only way we'd get Gregg to sit down with both of us. He said yes to my invitation without hesitation.

Though it was the first day of March, it was a shirt-sleeve day, one of those spring pre-cursors we get often in winter in my hometown. As always, I was doggedly optimistic. Gregg and I had always been closer than he and his dad had been. When push came to shove, he'd usually talk to me. These descriptions by his roommates were deeply disturbing, but surely he'd tell me what was going on. When Will and I showed up at his doorstep together, though, Gregg was furious. He wasn't expecting his dad, viewed him as "the enemy." He gave me his "What are you thinking?" look, only this time he was more agitated than confused. But he went with us, and we drove to a nearby corner grill where we could sit in a booth and have a rational conversation on neutral ground.

Gregg was smoking constantly, but that was the least of our worries. He'd lost weight, had dark circles under his eyes, and his skin was pale, as though he hadn't been out in sunlight for some time.

We'd hardly sat down and opened our menus, though, before Gregg jumped up and said, "I'm not gonna do this. I'm getting out of here." Stunned, Will and I followed Gregg and convinced him to get in the car so we could go back to his place and talk. He got in the back seat, we got in front, and we headed toward Gregg's place. As we were driving through the Fan, one of us said something, something innocuous like, "Gregg, what's going on with you?" and he jumped out of the car while it was moving, and ran. Will pulled over to the curb; neither of us had a clue what to do next. We were both scared speechless. I went to my mother's nearby and called John. Will needed to stay close by. He was unhinged, uncertain of where to go at that point. We'd communicate later. We had to do something. Gregg's roommates were gone for the weekend so we could move him out. I'd get John in town; we'd catch our breath, talk, and do something.

Up to this moment, this was the most bizarre behavior from Gregg that I'd seen with my own eyes, and it was unsettling in a deep soul way.

It felt unreal telling John, "Gregg jumped out of the car while Will was driving." John arrived within hours. We met at a neighborhood pub and talked; he and I knew this was serious, well beyond anger or self-absorption. Paired with what Will had reported from the roommates, we had to conclude that something was extremely wrong with Gregg. He needed help, way more help than Will and I could give him.

Will acted on his own next, though I would have agreed with what he did if he'd asked. Perhaps he worried I would have tried to stop him if he'd consulted me. I wouldn't have. After he'd left me after our fiasco with Gregg, Will went to his college roommate's home, Gregg's Godfather. He asked Denny to come with him. The two went back to Gregg's apartment to try to talk to him, but he refused to let them in. Gregg ranted things like, "You have no constitutional right to be here" and "You'd better go away before I call the police and have you arrested for trespassing," so they left. Will called Gregg's former male psychologist—Gregg wasn't in therapy at the time—and described what our son had done that morning, as well as his behavior in the past weeks with his roommates. The doctor told him to go to the police and swear out a TDO, Temporary Detaining Order. Gregg would be Green Warranted, or TDO-ed, by the police if he did not go willingly to a hospital with Will and Denny.

A city social worker who served as a Crisis Intervention Specialist went back with them. Two policemen waited on the sidewalk. Gregg came to the door for the social worker, and when he explained who he was and what the consequences were, Gregg let Will, Denny, and the social worker into the house. The social worker told him he could go willingly to the emergency room at MCV, where he would undoubtedly be admitted to the psychiatric ward, or he could be arrested and taken to jail where he would be evaluated by a judge for competence the next day. I wasn't there, but I know Gregg refused to admit himself and that the police had to come in, arrest him, and carry him to the station in handcuffs and shackles. I know that he screamed horrible curses at Will and Denny. I know for Will and Gregg, it was a life-changing moment.

Afterwards, Will called, talked to John, and described to him what had happened. John was one hundred percent sympathetic and assured him we would have agreed with his decision. I was sorry John hadn't helped him, that Will hadn't asked John to go with him, too, instead of Denny. I know Will didn't want me there, and he was right in that decision. I would have tried to get Gregg to go with the social worker to the hospital, but when he didn't, could I have tolerated seeing police carrying him away like that? Probably not. I do know John would have gone with Will. Despite everything that had happened, he loved Gregg like a son.

The next day was far worse. Will and Betti and John and I were "invited" to Gregg's commitment hearing in the city jail psychiatric lock-up. Will had asked Gregg's former psychologist to come, and even at such last-minute notice he'd agreed to be there. We were a sad family contingent in a nightmarish place. All I could see was grey; all I could smell was some strong cleaning product and mold.

Before we went back to Gregg's cellblock, where the officer planned to hold the proceeding, the jailer told us, "Your son's been lying on the mattress on the floor without moving or speaking since we brought him in." The social worker and psychiatrist had both tried to talk to him about his options and to describe the legal procedure he would face. In hushed tones, each told us he had not acknowledged their presence or indicated in any way that he knew where he was or what was going on around him.

The jailer spoke up, in a surprisingly gentle voice, "If you want, you can go back and try to talk to him. But . . . don't be shocked by what you see." The psychologist explained that if Gregg would admit himself to the MCV psychiatric ward, where the doctor had found a bed for him, it would be far better than if he was forcibly admitted to the state psychiatric facility outside Petersburg. There, once court committed, he would stay until released. That could be a week or a lifetime. Of course we'd try to talk to him.

Will and Betti went back first. They came out grey-faced, sadder than sad. He hadn't moved, hadn't spoken. John and I went in. Gregg was locked behind bars, on his stomach on an old ticked mattress, hands cuffed behind his back. We went into the cell and knelt next to him.

I talked to him. "Gregg, you've got to talk. You've got to help yourself, Boog. A judge is here. They're going to put you in a state hospital. If you don't speak up for yourself, you're going to lose your rights. You've got to talk." Not a blink. Not a move. Not a flicker of his eyes. He appeared catatonic to me. John tried. Nothing. We went back out shaking our heads no, unable to speak to one another or the others.

The sheriff was a kind man. He must have hated this part of his job. "I'll get so-and-so (another jailer, a giant of a man, as it turns out) in here. We'll drag your son out of the cell. The law says he has to be present at his hearing. He has to have the chance to speak in his own behalf. There's not enough room in the cell for all of us." Someone brought in chairs and formed a kind of semi-circle in front of the judge, a still, mousey-looking man who'd been waiting all this time. No one sat but him. The two officers went in and dragged Gregg out. He was still immobile. As one of the officers called us to order and we began to move to the chairs, Gregg turned and half sat up.

He began screaming. "Fuck you, Mother. Fuck you, Dad. Do you hear me? Fuck all of you!" The look on his face was primal, feral, full of hatred. I have never seen nor heard anything like it, but the only thing I can imagine that comes close is demonic possession. The Gregg I knew was not in this body. That was not his voice. He turned back around, lay back down, and never said another word during his commitment hearing.

The legal part was short. The judge had seen what he needed to see. There was no doubt this young man needed to be hospitalized. But he went through the formalities, speaking directly to Gregg's prone back. "Mr. Smith, are you having any thoughts of hurting yourself?" No answer. "Let the record show that Mr. Smith did not respond. Mr. Smith, are you having any thoughts of hurting others?" No answer. "Let the record show that Mr. Smith did not respond. Mr. Smith, have you recently been suffering delusions, which is hearing voices in your head, or hallucinations, which is seeing things which are not there?" No answer. "Let the record show he did not respond. Mr. Smith, would you be willing to check yourself into a hospital of your choosing to receive psychiatric assistance for the period of forty-eight hours?" No answer. "Let the record show he did not respond. I hereby commit Gregg Smith . . ." and that was it. We waited to sign the legal papers as witnesses. He would be taken by ambulance within no more than twelve hours to Eastern State Hospital where he would receive a complete psychiatric evaluation and work-up in no more than seventy-eight hours. At that time, the team of psychiatrists could choose to release him or hold him for treatment. There would be no value in calling prior to the end of that period. They would not be able to tell us anything.

We left all our names and numbers. Gregg's therapist stayed with us. What a wise, kind man. He told us his suspicion, "Gregg undoubtedly has some form of psychosis, which is likely an indicator of some type of schizophrenia. If that's the case, he'll respond quickly to medication, but he might require life-long treatment." He said Gregg had all the earmarks of schizophrenia, but it was a difficult diagnosis. We shouldn't expect a quick diagnosis or quick results. Newer medications were coming on the market, but people with a diagnosis in this spectrum often went off meds when they started being able to do "normal" things again, because they hated the side effects. But we should all wait and see. He couldn't say until we got the intake evaluation.

Everyone was in emotional shreds, partly because we'd been unable to talk Gregg into signing himself into MCV, which had a trial program going on at that very time dealing with treatment plans for adults with schizophrenia. We'd all heard the horror stories about state mental hospitals. But mostly because we'd seen a Gregg we didn't know existed. Or, more to the point, the Gregg we'd known wasn't there any longer. But for the time being it was out of our hands; we'd done the best we could.

Years later, while he was still ill but not psychotic, Gregg wrote a play, *Witch's Lament*, that he asked me to read. In it, the main character, Willy, is arrested and TOD'ed. I've included an excerpt from his play in the Appendix (APPENDIX I, item 1.) that demonstrates Gregg's view of that nightmarish series of events leading up to his hospitalization.

CHAPTER 8 -- INTO THE ABYSS

That day of the commitment hearing, part of me went into a dark abyss with Gregg, and neither of us has ever emerged the same again. That place, that experience, though in "real" time, it had a beginning and an end, will never end for me. Any notion I had that Gregg was going through a phase, was struggling for identity, was having a tough time finding his place in an unforgiving world was completely over. He was seriously mentally ill. I had no idea whether he'd ever "come back" to sanity, or even if he'd ever leave the hospital.

When I told my parents about Gregg's psychotic breakdown, they gave me some shocking news of their own. Gregg had stolen money from his grandfather's wallet. He'd forged a couple of checks on my mother's account. In all, he'd ripped them off for about six hundred dollars. Once when he was over, he'd gone across the street to the neighborhood drugstore and come back so "messed up" that he'd frightened them both. At the time, that corner was noted for its drug scene; they were sure he'd hooked up with a supplier. They hadn't told me any of this because they hadn't wanted me to worry. I was reeling.

As directed by the judge, I waited to call the hospital. When I did call, I was assigned a social worker. She would handle questions regarding hospital policies: visiting hours, who was permitted to visit, providing necessities for the patient, and all of the logistical information. Until "a patient" gave permission, no one at the hospital could or would even identify that he was admitted. Fortunately, she was able to tell me that my son was there; he had signed the permission form for me to speak to his doctors and to visit.

Via phone, the doctor gathered personal history information from me related to all aspects of Gregg's life. I withheld nothing. He told me that Gregg was heavily medicated and thus no longer psychotic, but the medication had serious kinetic side effects. From familiarity with the special education field, I knew what kinetic meant—related to the kinesthesiology system, or muscles—but I couldn't see how it related in this case. He explained that most of the anti-psychotic medications they used caused muscle dystonia, or stiffening. Facial affect, then, often appeared stiff and un-responsive. The patient was aware of the physical changes but unable to do anything about them. For some it was worse than others. Gregg was sleeping and eating. He would begin psycho-therapy within the week. It was too soon for a diagnosis. I told him that the psychologist suggested a schizoid-type disorder. He explained that he would not rule that out at this point, nor would he rule it in. It was a "difficult diagnosis"—I was to hear this phrase often in coming months—way too soon to tell. The process would not be fast.

In Gregg's play, *Witch's Lament*, he described the mental hospital where his character and alter ego Willy is committed (APPENDIX I, item 2.). In his view, often the medical staff was as "disturbed" as the patients they were treating.

I was working full-time teaching a five-class load at the community college. I was able to get away only on weekends. That first Sunday, I went to see Gregg alone. I took what I was allowed to take: white T-shirts, socks, cigarettes, and a pair of flip-flops. After I checked in at a glass-enclosed booth, I was directed to the day room where I would wait until he was roused by an orderly. Men shuffled around in pajamas. Mostly it was subdued, with lots of worn This End Up-style furniture and fake plants, people smoking, not many "civilians." I didn't like to see Gregg in my mind's eye in this place. I knew he hated it, and so did I, but the image cannot be erased. I couldn't look away.

He came shuffling down the hall in pajama bottoms and a kind of papery robe and T-shirt. He was slow, stiff, blank-faced. Like Frankenstein, I hated myself for thinking. I hugged him and he hugged back, hard, but neither of us cried. We sat and talked. His speech was slow. When I told him I brought cigarettes, he went to the desk and asked for them. He chain smoked, lighting one from the other since he couldn't have a lighter. An orderly stayed in the room. I thought Gregg would be angry and attack me for committing him, but he wasn't. I thought he would ask a lot of questions, but he didn't. I tend to over-talk when I'm nervous, so I rambled on about John and Miranda and our dogs, Jackson and Bianca. He contributed little, asked no questions. When I decided to go, he hugged me again, and I hugged back hard, but he didn't seem to mind me leaving, and I couldn't get out into the fresh air soon enough.

I felt like I was going to have a panic attack, so I took deep breaths in the car and tried to stay calm. This visit felt surreal, like I'd imagined it. I'd been inside the hospital no more than half an hour, but I was certain it had been at least two hours. Gregg wasn't himself, but he wasn't anybody else I knew either. The three-hour drive home felt like it took forever. I hated all this more than I've ever hated anything.

I didn't go back for at least two weeks. The doctor told me he'd been able to regulate Gregg's medicines, so he was no longer so zombie-like, and they'd begun psychotherapy, though getting him to open up was slow-going. He had no idea. It'd taken about seven years, by my count.

The next time I visited, Gregg was talking a lot, and much of what he was talking about was sex-related. He told me that the doctor was way too curious about his sex life. The questions about masturbation creeped him out. What did that have to do with anything? If I was to ask him, the doctor was the one who was a sicko. Now he was high-fiving the "brothers" who were in there with him; other patients who were the slightest bit lucid called him by name—"Wha's up, Gregg Man?" His face was more expressive (any expression at all would be more expressive), but the smiles were more like smirks, and his eyes weren't calm at all. They jumped continuously. He had focusing problems and complaints of blurred vision. He was glad to see me, he was glad I'd come, he didn't think he belonged there at all. I didn't stay much longer than half an hour this time either. It was too weird, unsettling, and scary. Different hadn't necessarily been better.

His dad went to visit him during evening hours. I was glad to hear this. Strangely enough, Gregg didn't express anger toward either of us. He didn't like the medicine. He wanted to get out. But Will and I weren't his targets for the time being. That was about the only good news. A social worker was assigned to help Gregg plan for release, and he took a sincere interest in Gregg's "re-entry," to the point of driving him around to look at suitable apartments. We still didn't have a diagnosis; the doctors would not say at that point that Gregg was suffering from paranoid schizophrenia, because the only psychotic episode anyone could document was the one surrounding the arrest. The closest thing to a diagnosis at that moment was schizo-affective disorder. Gregg would be released to the care of a mental health agency in a few more weeks. He would have to stay on medication and report for regular examinations. We were assured that many people with such a diagnosis led full lives. There was no medical reason he couldn't return to school once he was out of the hospital.

Gregg wanted to move back into the city, close to the college. Will thought that the temptation to return to his drinking/druggie ways was too likely in the inner city, that Gregg had too many "connections" there. Besides, the mental health services were far superior in the county. Until Gregg could be assured of a place to live, he could not leave the hospital. Will would provide for the apartment, but he refused to lease one inside the city. Meanwhile, Gregg needed to have some experiences with short-term release, going out for a few hours at a time on day passes. The social worker did some of this. I decided to take him out for an afternoon, too. I was scared, though. What if he became irrational? What if he tried to run away? We'd go out to eat and to a movie. Including driving to and from the hospital, that would cover the time he was allotted.

When I went to pick him up, he was dressed in his own clothes: khakis, a plaid shirt, and tennis shoes. He was a bit wrinkled and mussed but at least not in that helpless hospital garb. Still pale, he wasn't as stiff as he'd been a month earlier. He smiled, and he didn't say inappropriate sexual things. I detected definite improvement; he even demonstrated a sweetness I hadn't seen in quite a long time, spontaneously grabbing my hand, thanking me for coming to take him out. But somehow all the same features that had added up to a handsome young man only weeks before now formed the face of a person who appeared needy, off-kilter—well, crazy. He was like a Picasso version of himself that I couldn't quite focus into a natural whole.

I let him choose where we'd have lunch. He didn't have any grandiose request, just, "Could we go get a real pizza?" We went into town and ate pizza at a depressing mom and pop joint, then went to see *Good Will Hunting*. John and I had seen it. I'd described it to Gregg, and he thought that might be an okay choice. The portrayal of this super-intelligent outsider finding his way to health and the opportunity for a fulfilling life seemed like positive fodder for him as he looked at decisions about this next phase of his life. Still, it was odd sitting there with my own Will Hunting, wondering what he was thinking and how he was taking this. Afterward, as we drove back to the hospital, he said he'd liked the movie. He mostly wanted to talk about getting out and starting over, though, which struck me as positive. He wasn't psyched about moving into the county—he had his own reverse discrimination thing going about "preps" and "West Enders." Maybe he was afraid of running into old private school friends, unable to hide his setbacks compared to their successes, but he didn't say this. Still he was excited about being out, about being on his own, about going back to school. He hated the medication. He tried to describe it: "like having a screen between me and what I'm doing, like when I look in a mirror I'm seeing some monster/horror creep, not myself." But he'd do whatever it took to get out of the psych hospital. And he swore he'd never go back there again.

Scary as this off-grounds visit had been, this Gregg felt more like the little boy I'd known back before his teen years, like he'd time traveled backwards and gotten stuck around ten. None of that rawness, that edgy, sly meanness he'd demonstrated at the jail remained. I went home optimistic. As always, John tried to temper my enthusiasm. This time I got mad at him.

"I hate it when you do that. I'm the one who's been spending time with Gregg. He's nothing like he was before, at the jail. Why do you always have to be so negative about him?" My throat chokes up and I get teary when I'm mad, so I couldn't say much more. John assured me that he wasn't being a nay-sayer; he didn't want me to get my hopes too high, that was all. I needed to keep my expectations in check. Gregg was still a sick young man. That wasn't what I wanted to hear.

John and I planned to pick up Gregg on the day of his release. Will would have the key to his apartment, would deliver Gregg's furniture he'd kept in storage, and would arrange to get his car there. John and I would help him get the place unpacked and set up and take him grocery shopping. We'd be sure he had his meds, and we'd leave when he was ready for us to go.

My recollection of this day is quite different from Gregg's fictional version in his play, *Witch's Lament*. I was seeing his new place for the first time, and I was impressed with it. Will had found a sunny, one-bedroom garden apartment and stocked it with everything Gregg would need except food. John and I had brought some additional furniture and household goods, and we arranged the place to look homey and inviting. We hung pictures, made the bed, got the kitchen set up. Gregg and I went to the grocery store together while John wired the stereo components, and while it was slow going at the store, we talked about healthy eating and picked out soups and cheeses and the things he wanted. Per usual, I was acting chipper—perhaps falsely chipper, I must admit, but I'm noted for "making the best of a bad situation," as my grandmother always advised.

Perhaps in my cheeriness, I was missing signals from Gregg that he was afraid, that he feared loneliness, that he wondered if he was actually ready to be on his own. I can say I didn't pick up on this, and neither did John. Gregg has always played his cards close to his chest. When I asked if he had taken his medication, he was openly irritated for the first and only time that day, but I wasn't surprised. He was an adult, twenty-six years old, after all. At some point, John began to get antsy. We'd stayed longer than we'd planned, but I was having a hard time pulling away. I felt certain Gregg didn't want us to go. But the entire treatment team had said this was the right next step, so we left. (See APPENDIX, item 3.)

Gregg returned to VCU. His dad supported him, and he worked hard. He'd gotten glasses in the hospital for his blurred vision, and he began to look better than he had in some time, almost studious and calm. His apartment complex had a fitness gym, and he suggested he'd work out some. That Christmas we gave him a bike, which he'd wanted, so he could sometimes ride back and forth to school. It was a long haul, but he wanted to get his muscle tone back. This was important to him.

He continued to play guitar, but one of his greatest frustrations during this period was that the medicine prevented him from having the agility he once had in his hands and fingers, so he knew he played less competently. He also complained that because of the changes in his vision, he got headaches when he read.

Before (everything from this point on means "Before he was in the state hospital"), he could read and study for hours. This reduced attention span forced change in study habits. This loss angered him.

Mother's Day was a big celebration for all of us that year. Melanie's daughter Sasha had been born in February, on the 22nd. She had a rare blood disorder with petechiae all over her from head to toe at birth, and leukemia and hemophilia were the two first speculations by the neonatal specialists when they rushed her to neonatal intensive care. We didn't even get to hold her. In NICU, she had to have three platelet transfusions before her platelet factory kicked in and she was safe from brain hemorrhage. Luckily, her condition was not chronic, and she went home healthy two weeks later. I had gone from the hospital with Melanie and Sasha to the jail with Gregg; this was a harrowing convergence of events, but on Mother's Day in May, Sasha was Christened, and we had an enormous celebration at my mother's.

Gregg came, bringing cards for me and Betti and my mother. Each was chosen with care, and inside he'd written each one of us a personal, loving message. He hugged us all and was truly his sweet, younger self. He's pale and thin in the snapshots from that day, but the fact that he was with us is an important aspect of our sense of hope and blessings.

I saw another movie during this period that reminded me of Gregg. John, Miranda, and I had gone to D.C. to visit a close friend from our former teaching days. The adults went to see *A River Runs Through It*, with Brad Pitt in the starring role as a self-destructive, bright, handsome journalist. Gregg even resembled Pitt, and it was too much. At the end, when Pitt's family confronts his death, I started crying and couldn't stop. The lights came up, everyone left the theater, and I sat there and bawled in a way I hadn't wept since this all began. In the movie, I had looked at the path Gregg was on and all of my anxiety and worry and fear came pouring out. The others left me alone until I finished, and I left the theater leaning on John, unable to say a word.

School did not go well for Gregg, so he dropped out and found a job at Seven-Eleven. He got fired, he claimed for unfair accusations. In any case, he was miserable in Richmond. He wanted to go where the sun shone. He thought he'd sell his car and try California. No amount of advice on anyone's part could discourage him. He had no friends, no real prospects.

Whenever he ran into anyone he knew in Richmond, he felt low. They all had graduated from college, had professional jobs, and most were married. He hated running into those guys; it made him feel shameful. He'd always hated his West End apartment, never been comfortable there. A more relaxed lifestyle in the sun was bound to make him feel better, he thought. We had serious doubts, but Gregg was adamant. We had a good friend in California, in Venice Beach. He would help Gregg get set up.

At the time Miranda was in boarding school in Richmond. She'd gotten away from our country home as soon as she could. She loved her new situation, which was far more sophisticated and intellectually challenging. On her sixteenth birthday, Gregg had ridden his bike by to see her and to give her a CD. He'd always been her most loving sibling, but she had torturous mixed feelings about him and whatever was wrong with him. In part, she was afraid that she'd go "crazy," too. When required to write a narrative essay for English class, she poured out her conflicting feelings with amazing honesty. Gregg was her beloved brother, but he made her afraid and uneasy, too. (APPENDIX I, item 4.) I could never forget: Mental illness has an impact on the entire family, on every single person.

Although I couldn't agree with his choice, I came in to Richmond from the country that spring, and Miranda and I drove Gregg to the bus station. He'd sold his car, packed up what he'd need in a backpack, and stored his furniture at his dad's. We saw him off to California that day. I made him swear to me that he'd stay on his medication. He hugged us before he boarded the bus, confident that this was the right decision for him, sure he'd be fine once he took charge of his own destiny. Smiling, he waved goodbye, "Don't worry, Mom—be happy." A young man going west. None of us shared his optimism.

CHAPTER 9 -- MEXICO I

In California, Gregg bought a junk car he could use to hunt for work. He stayed with our friend Bill D., who was living in one of those guest quarters temporary situations. At first Gregg called often. When I talked to him, he sounded fine—the usual job search problems, but nothing bizarre. Then he had car trouble; in fact, he had car double trouble. Someone bumped him in L.A. traffic. He didn't get the name, insurance information, or license number, so he was furious about that. Then, running out of cash, he decided to sell the car. A guy paid him five hundred dollars, half of what he promised, and told him he'd bring the rest the next day. Gregg signed over the title, and he never heard from the guy again. This freaked him out, too.

He started calling us at odd times, saying he could hear people talking about him through the walls. I begged him to get his prescriptions filled, that I would send the money, but he insisted he didn't need that stuff, that it only messed him up. He made outlandish accusations: John and Jaison were out to get him. He knew that two girls from college had come to our house and told us terrible things about him, and we'd believed them, but they weren't true. John had no right to listen to them. He sent me the most hateful, distorted, disturbed letter I have ever read in my life, much of it about his sexual exploits.

Our friend Bill D. called us. Gregg wasn't leaving the apartment. He was sleeping a lot, eating a lot, out of money. He wasn't bathing, or he was bathing constantly. Talking to himself. Clearly he was psychotic again.

We sent Bill D. the money to put Gregg on a bus home. When he got back, disheveled and confused, we took him directly to the hospital, and a judge came in to evaluate him. This time, Gregg knew the right answers to their questions. No, he wasn't going to hurt anyone. No, he wasn't going to hurt himself. Of course he wasn't hearing anything that others didn't hear or seeing any things that others didn't see. He smirked and agreed to voluntarily commit himself. He was out in two days.

Will set him up in another apartment. He went back to mental health for his meds and re-entered school. I was incredulous that he could still get financial aid. How could that be? Why would they let him return? But they did. Will gave him a brand new, purple Ford truck with the proviso that he stay in school and stay on his medication. By this time, Melanie and Betti had had it with him. Once, when he called his dad's house, Betti told him to never call there again. From then on, he had to contact his father at work. Melanie said she couldn't ever forgive him, that the trouble and expense he was causing me and her dad were intolerable. She'd always hated that Prodigal Son parable in the Bible, and this was her reality now, and she was mad. Other people in his condition took their medication and led productive lives. He was still making bad choices, and she thought we were all too quick to help him when he wouldn't work to help himself. We chose to think that with treatment and medication, after his stint in a mental hospital and his failures in California, he'd "turn himself around."

That Christmas, Jaison came home with his fiancé Molly, a beautiful, brilliant young woman we immediately adored. Of course she'd meet all of Jaison's family on this trip, including Gregg. John was worried. We all went by Gregg's place to pick him up. John and I decided to take him some food and Christmas cookies. He'd insisted no one give him gifts, as he couldn't reciprocate. We had honored his wishes, but groceries were another matter, and all the children counted on my iced cut-out cookies at Christmas.

We'd called ahead, he'd agreed to see us, but when John went to the door, Gregg yelled out, "Wait outside. I'll be out in a minute." He came out, pulling on a wool cap. He was unshaved, scruffy. "Can we go for a cup of coffee at a café? How 'bout we take in those groceries when we get back?" He didn't invite us in.

Jaison jumped out of the car to hug him. "Greeeeggggg." Big smile, big bear hug. Gregg put his arms around his brother, but he was edgy. He smiled shyly as he met Molly. I figured he was embarrassed about his right-next-door to poverty lifestyle, his lack of success. We talked out in the parking lot, made plans for the next day.

Gregg ate a cookie—"Mom makes the best"—then he took the bags and went back inside. We'd been there for no more than ten minutes.

Christmas Day, Gregg refused to go to his dad's for lunch. My mother didn't invite him for dinner. Melanie, her husband, and their daughter Sasha would be there. We were forced to make choices we didn't want to make. Gregg had estranged Melanie and my mother didn't want to cause friction, so Gregg wasn't invited. Jaison, Molly, John, Miranda, and I ate brunch at Melanie's and then took Gregg out to Denny's, not talking about the fact that he wasn't going to be included in the traditional china and silver family dinner. We sat among the misfits and travelers, a fractured family with no place to be together. We squeezed into a long table/booth, everyone extra polite.

"Order whatever you want, Boog. Get the steak and eggs. I'm gonna have coffee and applesauce," I suggested, already full, striving to be perky and upbeat. We had our picture taken with Santa Claus. Gregg ate a hearty meal while we each drank coffee or soda and talked about any safe topic: the weather in Chicago where Jaison lived, Miranda's latest play at school, the dogs. It was a pathetic attempt at holiday cheer.

John and I got busy again with the second semester of school. We were "empty nesters," almost, with Miranda in boarding school. She was a budding actress, and we often came into town to see her in a production or attend a school event. We'd stay with Melanie; we couldn't get enough time with Sasha, who was thriving.

Gregg started off calling us often. Then his calls tapered off. Then he didn't call at all. I began to worry, and so did Will. I had friends at VCU. I contacted some to see if he'd been attending classes. He hadn't, for at least two weeks. Will got the apartment manager to let him into Gregg's place. It was worse than a pigsty, more like an indoor dump with empty beer bottles and fast food trash all over the floor and every surface. Gregg was gone.

We filled out a missing person's report, giving the police recent photographs and all the information that might be helpful finding him. Six weeks dragged by without a word. Will cleaned out Gregg's apartment. I'd called the police, Will would call the police, but they had nothing to report. During this period, I was unable to go to meeting on First Day (Sunday) mornings, mainly because my anxiety wouldn't allow me to sit in the silence for the hour. I began to pray at night like a child, "Please God, let Gregg be healthy and safe."

From all my religious education, from Baptists through Episcopalian to Quaker, I'd learned that prayers of petition were the "least spiritual," but I didn't know what else to do. I could find no other words. After days turned into weeks, I would add, "I can take anything, Lord, but I can't take not knowing where he is. I can't live with the not knowing." I knew to be careful what I prayed for, but having him gone forever felt like the one reality I wouldn't be able to bear.

Finally, after six weeks, I got a call at work one day from Will. They'd found Gregg in Cancun, Mexico. He was in jail, psychotic. The American consulate had called Will. We had approximately twenty-four hours to get our son out of a Mexican jail where he'd been incarcerated for stabbing a police officer. No doubt if he went before a Mexican court he'd be found guilty. We needed to get there right away. Their system required that Gregg be represented by a Mexican attorney.

By the time I got to the Richmond airport, Will had more information. Gregg had been arrested after a dance-club brawl. He told the American consulate who visited that he had not been involved in the fight, but they'd rounded up everyone in the club and taken them to jail. The next day they'd released him, but when they gave back his money belt, all of his cash and his passport were gone. He'd had three thousand dollars. When he complained about being fleeced, they'd told him to leave the jail immediately or they'd re-arrest him. Furious, he'd gone back to his youth hostel, gotten his backpack and two guitars (one his precious Martin) and gone out on the sidewalk and set them all on fire. Police were called. When one tried to restrain him, he'd pulled the guy's knife and flailed it around, at one point cutting his face. Gregg was arrested again, and this time he was awaiting trial. Will had hired a lawyer to go in to see him and assure him that we were on our way and would bring him home.

Will purchased his round-trip ticket plus a one-way for Gregg. I paid for my own but got on the plane in Richmond without a current passport. The ticket agent told me I could get a certificate of citizenship in the Atlanta airport if I had my driver's license and Will and I would swear to my citizenship. This would cost ten dollars and would serve to get me in and out of Mexico. We raced to do this and barely made our Atlanta flight to Mexico.

145

It was a frightening, dreamlike trip, amidst all the vacationers drinking tequila. I couldn't even read or work a crossword, my usual airplane diversions. What awaited us was even more bizarre and disturbing.

A tall, handsome, well-dressed Mexican attorney met our flight with one of those signs the tourist agencies use to identify clients. He was tanned, mustached, distinguished-looking.

"I want to see Gregg, please, now," I insisted, but he said we needed to do some paperwork first. Cordial, like we were talking about which type of wine I preferred. He whisked us to his office immediately, in his air-conditioned older-model luxury Lincoln. We drove through the lovely vacation area of salmon-colored buildings and restaurants with umbrellaed tables out front into narrow streets, parking in front of his storefront law office. We hesitated to get out, told him again we needed to see Gregg, to assure he was okay.

He assured us, "Please, patience, that isn't how these things work," ever smiling. Not to worry, he understood the time frame. We would need to trust him to handle this.

The office was strange. Everything in it, from candle-holders to lamps to furniture, had price tags. Smiling, he said his wife ran an import/export business. A desk for a secretary/receptionist was in the front room, but it was bare of the usual office supplies—no papers, no folders, no pens, no phone. He had a partner, but his partner was out. This was way too *Twilight Zone*.

In his office, what he needed to explain was the cost. The exchange of money. We needed to sign legal papers. Gregg was fine—he had visited him himself that morning, before our arrival—but in order to get depositions for his release from the two policemen involved—Two? We thought there was only one? Well, yes, but his partner had witnessed the crime and he, too, would need to file a deposition. It would be costly. Plus the one officer was still in the hospital with his wounds. Those bills, plus any doctor costs, would need to be paid. I was nauseous to the point of throwing up. John and I lived from paycheck to paycheck. Miranda's boarding school costs were astronomical. We each took a small amount from our pay for our retirement, but that was it. If I had any money in my bank account, after I'd paid for the round-trip ticket to Mexico, it would be a few hundred. This sum was in the thousands.

Will agreed to pay what was necessary. He had brought a sum of money with him. Full payment would be required in cash prior to Gregg's release. Will would need to have the rest wired. We both signed. The lawyer stood, grinned from ear to ear, and clapped his hands; he would now take us to see Gregg. Throughout this entire day, he was affable, as if he were selling a house or drawing up papers for a timeshare. The disconnect between his cheerfulness and our fear created even greater tension. Plus the heavy, relentless heat. All day I felt like I was going to faint or throw up at any moment.

We drove to a seedy part of Cancun—like some depression-era, small American town had been transplanted in Mexico. The unkempt houses were more like shacks, with only dirt in front. The only color I registered here was gray—none of the perky pastels in the tourist center. At no point were Will and I left to confer alone. As we were driving, the attorney gave Will his mobile phone to begin to make calls to his bank back home to have more money wired. It would have to be cash. He could only wire it in five thousand dollar increments. He would need three Western Union drafts. Three? With the cash he had brought? This was mind-boggling.

First we went to one three-story building which appeared only partially occupied. It reminded me of the news photos of war-torn buildings in Sarajevo. An apartment building, an office building, a government building? No signs identified it. Our escort told us to wait outside, no need to come in. He would go inside and policemen would bring Gregg out right away so we could talk to him. After that, we would take care of the legal business (read "money transfers") while he got the needed depositions and presented them to the court. Things would move quickly now. Gregg would be released to us and we could take him back to the United States.

"Simple, no?" There were more smiles, and he disappeared into the building.

For the first time, Will and I could confer.

Confused and scared I asked, "Does this seem legit to you? Do you think this guy is a shyster?" He'd talked to one of his former college roommates, a judge, before he'd left. He'd also spoken to two other attorneys. All of them described something quite similar to what was happening.

Grim, Will explained, "They all said get him out now, no matter what it costs." The figures he'd been given were actually higher than what we'd been told so far. But we had no bargaining chips. Back home, Betti was working on having the money wired. Getting all that cash in one afternoon wasn't easy. I told him I was sorry, there was no way I could put my hands on any money without selling our house. He never complained. It's amazing what he and his wife accomplished in such a short period. Neither of them could have slept. His only interest was getting Gregg home, no matter the cost.

He'd brought some medicine, some pills left over from Gregg's prescriptions. We would drug Gregg to get him on the plane, if that's what it took. He handed the pills to me, and we waited under a tree not much taller than Will. Talking wasn't easy for either of us.

Forty-five minutes later, the lawyer returned, smiling. "Gregg isn't here in this facility any longer. He was moved to another jail this morning."

"But why?" I almost cried.

"Who knows, these things happen." He shrugged and smiled. We would go there. It would only be a matter of minutes.

The second building was far grimmer than the first. It looked like an abandoned crack house. Mexican men in street clothes—tees or guayabera shirts and jeans—came and went. No one had on a uniform. They all wore guns crisscrossed on their chests, like the Mexican banditos in old cowboy movies. Again our attorney went inside, cautioning us to wait, Gregg would be right with us. On his way inside the building, he shook hands and talked with a couple of the other men. For once he wasn't smiling. After much hand gesturing and talking he walked back to us.

"Gregg is not here either, sorry to say. They will go for him." He gestured toward the men standing around. "He will be with us momentarily." I could tell that Will was feeling jerked around. His face looked like stone, like if he tried to say anything, he'd crack. The lawyer went inside. He didn't bother to make any excuse for why we weren't invited. We waited outside, under some scraggly tree. What were our choices? We didn't even have our own car.

In another half an hour, a Volkswagen Bug drove up, made a U-turn, and parked in front of the so-called jail. Two men hopped out of the front seats. The one from the passenger side pulled up his seat and reached into the rear. When he stood, he had chains in his hands, like he was pulling an animal. Then I saw the top of Gregg's head as the same man helped him out. My son stood and looked around. He was handcuffed. My knees buckled, just like they had when I first saw him in the bilirubin tank in NICU all those years before.

Gregg blinked as though the sun was blinding him, like someone who's been inside a cave. When he saw his dad and me, tears sprang into his eyes. He shuffled toward us, and I walked to meet him, arms outstretched. One of the guards undid his handcuffs. Gregg met me and hugged me hard.

"Take me home, Mama, please," he whispered.

"We're here to take you back, Gregg," I whispered back, still holding onto him, "but you've got to do exactly what we tell you to do, or it won't work. Swear you will."

"I will. Get me out of here."

I looked him in the eye, sending a silent plea and promise. Will walked over. Gregg's skin was grayish; he looked sick, terrified. His dark eyes were dull, like all the green had been washed out of them. His head had been shaved. When he'd left, his thick brown hair was long and wavy and beautiful.

"Take these pills." I handed him three. "Swallow them right now." He did.

Will told him that we had a plane ticket out of there for him, but he wasn't to say or do anything that might jeopardize his release. He'd probably have to go before a magistrate. He should be one hundred percent cooperative and respectful. We were doing everything they asked us to do, and he should do the same. This was our one chance. Will promised we'd get him out. Today, if possible. Otherwise, tomorrow.

We'd seen Gregg psychotic, but we'd never seen him pathetic and broken. The guards took him inside, while we waited for the attorney to come out. We didn't have anything to say to each other.

The lawyer eventually joined us and he was smiling. "I told you he was fine. Yes? We should go back to my office, so you can call and check on the funds," he said to Will. "While you do that, I'll get the depositions. Then we'll pick up the money and your troubles will be over." We asked him to check the airport, to see if we could get a flight out this evening if he was able to spring Gregg by then. He said he would.

I would have laughed at the "our troubles will be over" comment if I'd had any laughter in me. Back at the office, Will made numerous calls. Some of the money was on its way; Betti was getting the rest, and he could expect it before the banks closed. I was confused: What difference did the bank closing make? The lawyer explained that the "deal" would not be complete until he deposited all of the cash in some account. His legal account? Of course. In any case, we would need to pick up the cash at Western Union, go to the bank to deposit a portion of it, distribute the remainder to the parties involved, and then he would bring us Gregg. "No problem."

Will and I waited in the reception area until he got the call that all the money had been wired. Then we knocked on the lawyer's office door, and he came out immediately to drive us to Western Union. The line was as long as the ride lines at Disney World. He said no matter, took Will up to a window, and spoke to the teller. Somehow he was given preference. I sat in a chair out of the way. Will had to fill out information for three money transfers—no, he could not complete just one.

Time was tight. We had decided, while we waited for the last phone call, that we would leave that night if Gregg was turned over to us. Though our airplane tickets were for the first flight out in the morning, and we'd planned to stay in a motel out by the airport once we had him, he was in such bad shape that we wanted to get him out immediately.

Once Will had the cash, he gave it all to the lawyer, all fifteen thousand dollars, plus whatever he'd given him earlier. We walked out to the sidewalk, and the tall Mexican lawyer told us we were to wait right there, he would hurry to the bank, make the needed payments, and return in an hour with our son. Before we could object, he was gone.

Will and I looked at one another. "We should have gone with him," I said.

"I know," he answered.

"He has all the money, doesn't he?"

"Yeah. But we know his name."

I tried to remember if a name was on his office door. I couldn't picture it. I couldn't remember the street address, either. We'd driven around so much, I had no idea where we were in relation to his office. We hadn't driven far to Western Union from there. I did remember that. Neither of us said the obvious: What if he'd driven off with the money? What would we do then? We stood on a street corner in Cancun, the light fading, watching buses crammed with Mexican day laborers go by. Scared and sad, I just stood there.

Finally Will said, "Are you hungry?"

For the first time, I realized we hadn't eaten all day. "No, I'm not. I don't think I could eat anything."

"Me either." He paced back and forth. He checked his watch, but only a few minutes had passed. "I need to walk. I can't just wait here."

"Okay." I couldn't stand there by myself. We started off. I think he wanted to try to back track to the law office as much as he wanted to burn off nervous energy. I walked along beside him, and sure enough, we came to the street where the lawyer had his office. We walked down it. The attorney's car wasn't there. No lights were on. But at least we'd been able to find it and commit the street name to memory.

We kept on walking quite a bit. We came to a lot of shops that I didn't remember passing earlier. The evening got darker until finally I suggested we go back. We tried to retrace our steps, but neither of us was certain which way to go. I began to feel panicky but I made myself stay calm.

Will finally said, "Let's get a cab."

"What do we tell the driver?"

"Western Union."

Right. That made sense. We'd been told not to take taxis except those at the hotels or motels, but we really didn't have a choice at that moment. Besides, what if the lawyer had come back and we'd missed him? Will tried to flag a few cabs, but none stopped. We kept walking, and finally we found one parked at the end of a block. Will asked him to take us to Western Union.

"Si, si," he told us, opening the back doors. I was scared to death, but I got in. The driver U-turned and drove only four or five blocks before he let us off in front of the right building. Will paid him and we got out on an empty sidewalk. It was night, all the businesses were closed, and we were alone. There was nothing to do but wait.

Within fifteen minutes, the lawyer's car drove up. Someone else was driving, a man not dressed like an attorney. The lawyer was riding shotgun.

"Jump in, por favor," he yelled. "We will meet your boy in just a few minutes." Will and I scrambled into the back seat, and the car squealed away from the curb. We drove to a busy area with lots of lights and shops; this must have been close to where we'd just been, but it was far glitzier. The tourist Cancun. We pulled up to a curb and waited. A cab drove up, Gregg jumped from the back seat, our lawyer pushed him into the back seat with us, and we took off again.

"Gregg, you don't have on any shoes." I reached over Will for Gregg's hand.

"Assholes took my tennis shoes," he said. Across his dad's lap he squeezed my hand. "Gave me back my wallet, empty, and my backpack, empty, and took my goddamn tennis shoes."

Will whispered to him, "Shut the hell up." He did.

The lawyer leaned over his seat smiling as though he'd won the lottery. Come to think of it, I guess he did. "We got back his belongings and his passport. That was quite fortunate."

The driver was speeding like a maniac, but I didn't say another word. The lawyer continued.

"We have just enough time to get to the airport. I have called ahead to change your flight, and they have tickets waiting, but you must pay the extra change fee. We have to be fast."

"What about shoes? Will they let him on barefoot?" I had to ask. I didn't want to get there and be turned away.

"Don't worry about it, Charlotte," Will said, but the driver pulled to a stop at the next corner, so I jumped out, ran into a gift shop, and bought Gregg a pair of flip-flops. We raced along through the night, and when we pulled up to the curb at the airport, the lawyer jumped out with us to help us make the final arrangements for our flight out.

"The least I can do," he insisted, still smiling. He ran ahead of us to the Air Mexico desk. I gave Will my ticket, and he jogged alongside the attorney, Gregg and I bringing up the rear. We had to go through customs; we didn't have bags, but we had to show our passports. Gregg and Will gave the inspector their passports. He lingered over my certificate of citizenship, made me show my driver's license, but finally he stamped my papers and let me through the gate.

"Get me a cigarette, Mom. I need a cigarette," Gregg was begging as I tried to hurry him along.

"We've got to run, Gregg. Come on. If we don't make this flight, we're gonna have to spend the night here." It was like he didn't have a fast speed any more. Maybe the medicine I'd given him had calmed him down too much.

When we caught up to Will, he was making the ticket adjustments. I tried to give him my credit card, but he insisted I stay close to Gregg, who'd started wandering up to people. I went after him. He was trying to bum cigarettes. Someone gave him one; he lit it and smiled.

"Come on, Gregg. We've got to go to the gate." I could see Will saying goodbye to the attorney, shaking his hand. I guess he had to. He had gotten us Gregg.

"Damn, Mom, look at all these sand niggers." Gregg started laughing.

I could barely speak. Gregg, spouting racist slurs? He'd never demonstrated an ounce of bigotry his entire life; his one and only high school love, for two years, was mixed race. How much lower could he stoop? Obviously he was psychotic.

"Shut up, I mean it. If you act up, you're gonna get thrown back in jail."

He kept on grinning a goofy, I've-got-a-secret grin, but at least he stopped talking.

Will caught up to us. "This flight's gonna board in about ten minutes. It'll be longer, cause we have to go through Mexico City instead of direct."

I didn't care; as long as we could get back to the U.S., I'd be happy. They could throw us off in Atlanta for all I cared.

"Hey Dad, did you see all the sand niggers?" Gregg said, grinning.

"Shut up, Gregg. I mean it. Shut up!" Will and I looked at one another, scared and despairing. We were the people who never said shut up, but Gregg was saying things we couldn't imagine him saying because they were so offensive.

We had to get out of Mexico. We boarded; none of us were sitting together, but we'd been lucky to get on the flight at all. Thank heaven Gregg went to sleep. I don't think he even woke up when we stopped for a layover in Mexico City. When we took off for Atlanta, I decided to try to sleep, too. The passengers had thinned out, I could stretch out across three seats, and after I said a prayer of thanks, I closed my eyes.

When I woke in the morning, the flight attendant served coffee and said we were only about an hour or so from landing in Atlanta. A couple of elderly Frenchmen a few seats back were talking, somewhat loud, as old people will. Otherwise the cabin was quiet. Will moved up and we spoke quietly, briefly, about what to do next after our final hop to Richmond. Betti had arranged to leave a car for him at the airport. We would drive Gregg directly to St. Mary's as soon as we landed in Richmond.

As we whispered, all of a sudden we heard someone scream, "Shut up, just shut the fuck up." We looked up. Gregg was standing, glaring back in the direction of the two old men, murder in his eyes. I had no idea what to do, but as fast as he'd stood, he lay back down again and didn't make another sound until we shuffled him from that plane to the small one taking us back to Richmond, his dad whispering the whole time, "Just be quiet, Gregg. Don't say a word. You hear me. Don't say a word." I didn't care anymore about how tired I was or how confused or how frightened. We were going to get Gregg into the hospital, get him back into treatment. Maybe this time he'd hit the bricks hard enough, as that admissions director in Maine had advised those few years back. Maybe this time he'd had enough. I certainly had.

CHAPTER 10 – HOW BAD?

On the twenty-minute ride to the hospital, Gregg talked about Mexico. The sedating impact of the mega-dose of anti-psychotic I'd given him was wearing off, and he rambled on non-stop. The jail cell in Cancun just had one window, up toward the ceiling. It was the only air and light for about twenty-some men. A hole in the middle of the cement floor acted as a toilet for all of them. The men crouched on that floor all day, mostly in the dark, and slept on it at night without so much as a blanket. He didn't have any medicine; he went a little crazy. At night, rats and roaches crawled all over the place. His skin crawled all the time. Really crawled. They were given water, some bread, and beans. He'd been moved from place to place, he had no idea why or how many times. All of the cells were like that. He'd been in hell.

When we got to St. Mary's, he balked. He didn't want to go in. Will and I talked him into it, assuring him that this was the only place he'd be safe, so he made every effort to act calm, but he was jumping out of his skin. Right away, the physician on duty notified the county mental health officials who'd worked with him most recently. They agreed to send over a crisis team, to talk to him about committing himself for treatment. Two policemen arrived quickly; that's standard operating procedure when there's a "mental" patient involved, I've learned. They were bored and a bit embarrassed. We waited, thinking the crisis team would arrive any minute. Half an hour. An hour. Gregg became increasingly restless and argumentative. Whenever a policeman or nurse checked on him, he'd sneer. He began to talk in a rambling way about his rights. I tried to stay in the treatment room with him, but he didn't want me in there, so I paced the halls. At one point, Will asked him what had happened to the new truck he'd given him. Defensive, Gregg said he'd pawned it in Florida, he couldn't remember where. The ticket had been in his wallet, but the Mexican police had cleaned him out. He'd meant to go back and get it, but he hadn't.

I lost track of everything that happened in that emergency room, of much of what he told us; it was all so sordid, and I was so numb and exhausted from the round-trip to Mexico to rescue him. It took hours for the team to get to the hospital, causing me to question my understanding of the words, "emergency" and "crisis." At some point, Gregg began to get more physically agitated, then recalcitrant, finally verbally abusive, until the nurses called the police into his room and he was handcuffed to the bed. He raved about "police brutality" and "fuckin' lyin' parents" and America being no better than Mexico. By then no one could reason with him. Again, he was TDO-ed. Since he couldn't commit himself voluntarily, they wouldn't let him out. In the hours he'd been in the so-called emergency room, he'd gone from subdued and scared to full-blown psychotic and raving.

Eventually Gregg was sent to a brand new dual treatment program for men with drug abuse problems and mental illness. This most recent Mexican incident, as well as his calls from California, were enough for the mental health professionals to make a clear diagnosis: paranoid schizophrenia. Finally, I thought, Gregg's condition is clear-cut, the mental health professionals and psychiatrists know what medication regimen works best, and he's assigned to a place that can DO something. Surely we were finally on our path to treatment and cure and a normal life. It had taken more than ten years.

Oddly enough, this almost new facility was directly across the street from the now-closed P.I.R. where Gregg had been hospitalized at seventeen. This in-patient program was designed on a kind of tough love/AA regimen. To gain privileges, the men had to earn them. Former patients were in charge, though psychologists and a medical team supervised the individual treatment and group interaction. Once again on daily medication, Gregg at first resisted any sort of therapeutic assistance, not necessarily belligerent, but certainly stubborn. He'd sleep past meals and scheduled meetings, do his assigned chores slower than flowing mud, and refuse to speak in group sessions. But eventually, to gain visitation rights and then outside passes, he cooperated.

I visited as often as I could, and when he could go out, I'd take him out for coffee or a meal. He was rational but confused— not a zombie like other times he'd been medicated, but still dazed and "off." Why did he always get caught? Didn't I know that Melanie and Jaison had been drinking and sneaking around while they were in high school, too? How come I hadn't come down on them? I reminded him of Melanie's yearbook describing her as "Most Grounded" in the Senior Superlatives, and that Jaison was sent to live with his mother for a year because he'd refused to abide by our rules, but Gregg couldn't accept those as legitimate comparisons. Somehow in his version, everyone, especially his father, had been harder on him, kinder to the other children. I tried to be reasonable and straightforward, but John and I became targets for his perceived unjust treatment as a child. When I'd leave him, I'd be exhausted, full of self-doubt and sadness. Should I just accept his truth, would that be more helpful? I had no idea. He'd tell me that the "brothers" inside kept telling him he was lucky to have a mama who would visit him, and he needed to treat me with respect, but each time I'd come to see him, we'd start out well and end up bickering, stirring around in the past. This treatment team didn't talk to me. I told myself that this was part of the evolution of his program: first he had to get out all the anger and crap. Only then could he move forward. Moms are safe targets. Still, part of me accepted his criticism. Certainly I'd made mistakes, though I told myself over and over that I hadn't made my mistakes out of neglect or lack of caring or ill intent. I'd been ignorant at times, overwhelmed at times, working through my own mental health and marriage troubles at times, but I'd never knowingly ignored Gregg or his problems.

After almost two months, Gregg was released in better shape than he'd been in for years. I am certain of this. He was clean. He was on medication. While it had ill effects, he did not have that crazed appearance or flat look resulting from other anti-psychotics. He moved into a third-floor apartment above a lovely family in the north-side of Richmond. For the first time in I couldn't say how long, he was polite and thoughtful. The landlord family liked him. He worked and took college classes. While his eyes still bothered him, blurring due to the meds, he could handle a light reading load. Will gave him a computer, which he could use to write. He began to work on a screenplay.

On Thanksgiving, we all gathered at Mother's. Gregg came for dinner, a silver/china/crystal formal affair. He and my younger brother, Victor, who is reclusive, got into a political diatribe at the table. To tell the truth, this upset my parents and John, but it didn't bother me that much. We always got into political disputes when we got together. Perhaps this had been more heated than usual, perhaps Victor and Gregg had been a bit more fiery than was customary, but both of them could be hotheads.

I guess part of me was thinking that Gregg speaking up was a sign of mental health, not mental deviance. He still complained to me about the way other family members had treated him, how Melanie had lived only blocks away from him when he was in the Fan but wouldn't even invite him over to look at a football game or visit his niece. How Jaison rarely called, and when he did it was to give Gregg grief if he teased his fiancée. Since when couldn't Jaison take a joke? Gregg never accepted the fact that his rude comments and lack of manners made people ill at ease or downright angry. He still couldn't sort appropriate from inappropriate. That wasn't a good sign, but I was willing to take slow progress rather than insanity.

In her senior year, Miranda wrote a research project on schizophrenia for her ethics class. She called to interview me as part of her research. Later, she told me how difficult it was to do the presentation part of the project before her class, and how complimentary the teacher was regarding her understanding and compassion. (APPENDIX I, item 5.)

When Miranda graduated, Gregg came to the ceremony in coat and tie. Everyone in our family was there: Jaison and Molly from Chicago, Melanie and Sasha (she and her husband were separated), my parents, John and I. Gregg, pale and nervous, greeted us and agreed to a few pictures, but he sat alone. When Miranda received the school's Drama Award, all of us cheered. Gregg came to Mother's afterward for the celebration in Miranda's honor but didn't stay long. It was clear he was exhausted and ill at ease, but he'd made the effort. I learned later that he gave Miranda a letter of advice as her graduation gift, speaking with honesty about his own failings and lost opportunities, warning her of the dangers of drugs and alcohol. None of us knew that this would be the last family event he would attend for some time.

Gregg is a gifted writer. All through his schooling, he had been praised for his math brilliance, but he was equally good at written expression, though this was a talent he'd never particularly valued up to that point. Since his first hospitalization, he'd talked to me often about writing a screenplay. He wanted information about format, characterization. Once we met at the public library to look up information on the web. He persevered at this, the first thing he'd been motivated to do on his own in so long. He wanted my advice, but he didn't want to show me anything he'd written until he was finished. I knew the main character was named Willy; I knew he struggled with mental illness. I was fairly certain that the other characters had been shaped from family members. Aside from this, I was in the dark. But I was thrilled—Gregg had a substantive project, a personal passion.

About this time, John and I moved from Rockbridge County to Lynchburg. John was done with our "Walden Pond" thing, as he called it, plus he was tired of commuting. A neighbor had shot our puppy (he lived). We'd tried to purchase the field next door when our friend down the road put it up for sale. We made a fair offer, but he sold it to someone else for $500 more, and the new owner moved a double wide onto it. We decided to move closer to John's college. I'd find work teaching. If need be, I could commute for a while. Gregg told us he was unhappy we'd left Goshen. He found the country more "peaceful," the people less "phony," but he was no longer living with us so wasn't part of our decision-making.

Gregg decided to take guitar lessons again, too, another choice that made me optimistic about his increasing mental health. I helped him buy another guitar, not a Martin like the one he had treasured but smashed and burned in Mexico, but a more modest starter guitar. He took private lessons at a guitar shop. He dropped school, deciding it wasn't for him, and I couldn't disagree. He began to work as a waiter, which concerned me. Even under the best of circumstances, when he was trying hard, Gregg was slow of speech and slack of movement on his anti-psychotic cocktail. Plus he had developed a short fuse. Waiting tables in a busy restaurant sounded like a prescription for failure. And it was. When he was fired, he went out and got a job bussing tables. He quit this one over an argument with one of the waiters who wouldn't tip him out because he was too slow. Then he started washing dishes, which scared me. My mother managed restaurants and private clubs for years. She'd told me that kitchen staff are hard to keep, and often people who do menial kitchen work have drug and alcohol problems. I worried that this environment would be too tempting for Gregg.

He moved again to a house on Churchill with "friends" he'd made through some of his employment experiences. I went to see the house. These two guys had good steady jobs—one worked in computers—and the house was actually quite nice, though a "fixer-upper." They wanted a boarder in order to make extra money to do repairs on the place. I could see why Gregg liked it there, and the young men were in no way slackers or druggies as I'd feared. He continued writing his play and got work prepping salads in a kitchen. One month he called in a panic asking for rent money. Though John opposed it, we compromised and I gave it to him as a loan. Gregg had never really asked us for anything. I'd lent him money to help him out over a rough patch this one time. He'd been jumping from job to job, but he was working. When he was in the treatment center, the social worker there had filed for some back disability; he was due an award. When he got it, he'd pay us back, and he'd pay Nanny and Pawpie the money he'd stolen, too. For a while, this new arrangement went well. We talked often on the phone, I'd see him on occasion, and I had the impression he was getting his life on track.

Over time, the phone calls became strange. Gregg would laugh at things that weren't funny. He'd tell me sexual jokes that made me uncomfortable. I asked him if he was smoking pot again; he was. I asked him if he was still working; he wasn't. What was he doing for money? He'd set aside a bit, like six hundred dollars. Didn't he owe rent? Yeah, this would get him by for a couple of months. The guys didn't mind if he ate their food. They'd invited him to have steak dinner with them once a while back; he'd get them a steak one night, too. It would be cool. I told him to stay off the pot. He couldn't use it with the anti-psychotic medication. Weren't they testing his blood at the mental health clinic? Naw, when he went in for his monthly sit down, they just asked if he was using and he told them he wasn't. No blood tests during his check-up, no random testing either. I insisted that smoking pot was using; he insisted it wasn't. I begged him to clean up his act, pay his rent so he could stay put. He promised he would.

The phone calls became even more bizarre. He was locking himself in his room. One of the guys had a dog who barked all the time. This was getting on his last nerve. He was behind one month's rent, but so what? They wouldn't kick him out. They liked him. Hell, if they did, he'd just "go homeless." He thought this was hilarious. Besides, he still had a couple hundred. He'd give the guys that and they'd let him stay and catch up.

I could tell he was stoned. I told him to get clean, to go out and find work. He said he didn't have a car. I asked about his bike. He hadn't had that for a while; he couldn't remember what had happened to it. I tried to prompt him: he was on the city bus line; he could get a newspaper, circle some jobs; go out on the bus and job hunt. Naw, he could walk around the neighborhood and try to get work if he decided to do that. Besides, these guys were cool. They'd given him some pot before. He'd bought some and shared it. They wouldn't kick him out.

At some point during this period, he tried panhandling for money, sitting in front of a convenience store playing guitar with his hat out. He gave that up when he traded insults with someone who told him to get a life and then pulled a gun on him. As Gregg told it to me, he taunted the guy, saying he wouldn't pull the trigger, so the guy shot at him, missed, and chased him back to his house where he shot at him again. He was avoiding his roommates. They were both gone all day, working, and even if they threw him out, he wouldn't mind being homeless. What was the big deal? He laughed, despite my attempts to coax him back to reality.

The next month, he called and asked if he could come stay with us until he got on his feet. He'd been booted for non-payment of rent. I had to tell him no. He got furious. I reminded him I'd nagged him to get work before his money ran out. What the hell difference did that make? I was the mom. He was getting thrown out of his place. He didn't have anywhere to go. He didn't have any money. Did I mean to say that I was going to let him go out on the street? I wouldn't even let him come and stay a little while, a coupla weeks? I had an extra bedroom, plenty of food, money to live on, and I wouldn't share that with my own son, a son who was in trouble?

What the hell kind of mother was I?

He pushed all my buttons, but I wouldn't relent. John put his foot down. He'd told me that once we loaned Gregg money he couldn't come to visit until he'd made up a payment plan and started paying it back. Plus he was doing drugs again. This scared me to the bone, but I knew John was right. When I told Gregg this, he went ballistic. John always hated him, we had all that money, what had we ever done for him? I had no choice. John had said he couldn't come, and that was that. So Gregg blamed me when he went out on the street. I felt an enormous amount of guilt despite the fact that he'd foreseen this eventuality and laughed about it, done nothing to prevent it. He was a grown man who had to live by his choices, and I couldn't be his safety net this time or I'd be enabling the drugs and unemployment, but that decision tore me to pieces. The saying goes, "Home is the place that, when you go there they have to let you in." I wasn't letting him in. I wasn't his home any longer.

My mother allowed Gregg to store some of his belongings in her basement. She called me upset because I hadn't given Gregg a helping hand. Did I realize that he was homeless, that he had no money to live on, that he needed a haircut? Yes, I knew all that. How could I turn him away? I had to. Despite her criticism of my parenting—a scab that her attacks always tore wide open—I held my ground. I told her she was NOT to let him stay there. My parents are elderly; he'd stolen from them before, and I knew he was on drugs again. Mother assured me that Pawpie wouldn't let him stay there, anyway. She admitted they were afraid of him. But they would give him some money and drive him to my younger brother's. I made her promise that she wouldn't give him more than a twenty, since if she did, she'd in all likelihood be buying his drugs. My brother Victor lived alone in a sparse one-bedroom apartment. I could not imagine that he could tolerate Gregg, especially in the condition my son was in at the moment. My preference was for him to go to mental health, tell them he was using again, and seek in-patient treatment. He assured me he'd die before he'd do that again. My mother promised me that she'd take my son for a haircut, take him out to eat, and drop him at my brother's with twenty dollars in his pocket. John was right. Gregg had found a way to take care of himself. He'd mooch.

He stayed with Victor a while, which was hard on both of them. My brother had never married, never had children, lived alone purposefully on his savings, owning little. Gregg ate all Victor's food, left his dirty dishes in the sink, and slept on the sofa around the clock. In essence, he appropriated Victor's living space with no effort at consideration or gratitude.

My brother tolerated it as long as he could; even he, usually non-judgmental, asked why, as Gregg's mother, I wasn't doing something for him myself? Why weren't Will and I shouldering the responsibility? But what could I do? Mental health services wouldn't even talk to me any longer. This time Gregg had refused to sign a waiver of confidentiality, refusing giving them permission to tell me about him or any treatment he was getting. I knew he needed hospitalization, but I had no way to force it, except to refuse to let him come stay with us.

Gregg moved out of Victor's after a couple of weeks to a crack house in a section of Churchill I'd never even driven through in all my years in Richmond. He called me to tell me he had a place and he was working washing dishes again. Will loaned him an old farm truck to get around. He was taking his medicine, he insisted, trying to get back on his feet. I came into town and picked him up to go out to supper. It was a disturbing meal. We had to wait at the bar for our table. I ordered sparkling water, he ordered a beer. I told him I wouldn't pay for any alcohol for him, and he laughed and said he'd pay for his own beer and did. As we sat at the bar, he described the heroin addict who lived across the hall and the "uptown" rich girl he dated who liked him to abuse her. I was sickened. We moved to a table, and when my food came, a lamb dish I'd ordered, he began to describe in graphic, grisly detail the slaughter of a lamb, complete with gestures, laughing, and grinning. I asked him to please change the subject, he was ruining my meal. The hackles of my neck were up: inappropriate remarks, laughter out of context, these were red flags. Chastened, he apologized and moved on to the next topic without any sense that I had become truly uncomfortable in his presence. He told me he was sending me his play and asked if I'd type it on the computer in the correct format and make a diskette for him. He wanted to submit it to contests and agents. Would I help him? He ate with gusto, talked with animation. I was confused, upset, and could hardly wait to let him off again at his slum apartment.

He did send a copy of his manuscript, and while it was bizarre in ways, it showed promise. Clearly he could write and develop a character, and he had a strong sense of pace. His central character Willy, a mentally ill drop-out, was compelling. The graphic sex scenes and visitations by a succubus and thinly veiled portrayals of family members upset me. I transcribed *Witch's Lament* and told him I'd send suggestions for improvement. But by then he was arrested.

Will called to tell us that Gregg had been picked up for trying to sell drugs in a drug-free zone on the VCU campus. He went before a judge who recognized his last name; the judge recused himself but called Will from chambers to tell him what was going on and to assure him that he'd do what he could to help, but Gregg was in some serious hot water.

Dear Lord, How bad could things get? Gregg had had every treatment chance possible, and now he was in jail for selling drugs? I rushed to Richmond. His story was even more twisted than usual. He was out with a prostitute (a prostitute? What about HIV?); they'd wanted some drugs. Gregg and the addict across the hall made up some gel-tabs with Jell-O to sell for quick cash. They thought it was funny to scam the druggies. He'd gone to campus to try to peddle the gel-caps as some sort of upper. He'd approached two young men who said they'd be back with money but instead directed the campus police to him. The prostitute made off with his junk truck. When he was arraigned, the new judge permitted him to leave on his own recognizance, an unheard of break, as long as Will signed that he would assure Gregg would return for trial. Will had talked to Gregg about the importance of cleaning himself up for court, of taking advantage of this unbelievable opportunity to stay out of jail.

I got to town and took him out to eat, reenforcing what Will told him, to get some presentable clothes for him, and to assure myself that he was clean and sober and wouldn't end up in jail as a convicted felon. When I talked to him, he was truly scared to death. During his one night in jail he'd been propositioned by a far bigger, tougher street hustler. While Gregg is strong as an ox, he's small. Two men could overpower him. He didn't want to go to prison.

What happened next is inexplicable. Gregg went in for his drug testing as part of his release until his case was litigated, and his urine was filthy with cocaine. He was put into the city lock-up until his hearing. How had that happened? I'd seen him the night before, and he'd promised me he'd stay clean. Will and I were both stupefied. Prison appeared inevitable. Will refused to pay for Gregg's attorney now, and I couldn't blame him. The court appointed a lawyer, and Gregg would remain in the city jail until his court date.

Melanie was a practicing corporate attorney, and we didn't turn to her for legal advice related to Gregg's charges, but I did talk to her for information regarding legal proceedings. Crime was not part of her work, but she could call some friends who worked in prosecution and tell us what was likely to happen. Her disdain for Gregg and his increasingly disgusting behaviors and lifestyle only hardened. But she supported me and her father without fail, always listening and trying to boost me through this confusing, heart-breaking time. Miranda was out of state in college, so we didn't fill her in on all the tawdry details about her brother, thinking we'd tell her the outcome once Gregg had his trial and we knew the final determination.

Gregg asked me to come to his hearing, and I told him I would. His dad wouldn't. Who could expect him to do more than he had already? He'd given Gregg a legal life preserver and his son had betrayed him. Melanie insisted on going with me. I told her she didn't need to, but she thought I needed an ally, and despite her feelings about Gregg, she wanted to there to support me. My rock. John was working, so he couldn't be there. I met Gregg's attorney. She was sharp and businesslike but hurried and harried. However, she was optimistic. The first day was only a formality; his case would be sent to a higher court. It was good that I was present; perhaps the judge would release him until the next hearing if I was willing to certify that he would show up. Given his mental illness, his lack of a prior criminal record, and the expected outcome of the substance test (Jell-O, not a controlled illegal substance), she was hopeful he'd eventually get supervised probation. A social worker was trying to find a placement for him. Meanwhile, he could stay a certain number of days at the Salvation Army Men's Shelter downtown on an emergency basis. If a bed became available and he stayed clean, that would be the best situation for him until his actual trial.

Criminal court is a poor commentary on human nature. Name after name was called for drug offenses, soliciting for prostitution, breaking probation, and parole violations. When Gregg came in in an orange jail jumpsuit led by an armed guard, I was near my breaking point. How had he brought himself down to this? His attorney told the judge that his mother was present, and he looked around the courtroom, smiled, and invited me to come forward. I stood there as he read from the papers the clerk handed him regarding Gregg's crimes. He asked each attorney some questions. They agreed to what the judge proposed.

He spoke directly to me. "Ms. Morgan, are you Gregg's mother?" I nodded. "Are you willing to vouch for your son, Gregg Smith, and to assure the court that he will appear on the date the clerk assigns for his trial for these crimes in the general court?"

"Yes, sir." He spoke to Gregg, telling him he was a fortunate young man to have a mother to speak ion his behalf, and he expected to see him in such and such a court on such and such a date at such and such a time. Gregg answered respectfully, and he went in the back again to change and retrieve his wallet. I don't know how my legs carried me back down the aisle. Melanie hugged me and left to get back to work.

Outside, as Gregg and I walked to my car through the rain, he thanked me and promised he'd get straight this time. He wasn't allowed to go back to the slum house he'd lived in formerly. When his father had gone to clean it out, his belongings were trashed anyway. It was hard for Will to determine what was Gregg's messy lifestyle and what was vandalism, but his computer was gone, as well as some of his good clothes and expensive college texts. The addict neighbor had moved out. Gregg was certain that he and his girlfriend had stolen his computer and his expensive winter jacket to sell for drugs. I had a garbage bag of his clothes in the backseat that Will had given me. Gregg wanted me to take him to get some shoes and a few necessities at Goodwill—he didn't want me spending much money—and a carton of cigarettes, and he'd be fine. That's exactly what we did, but I still felt like I was in somebody else's life and I wanted out. I'd picked up my son at jail, driven him to a thrift store to get shoes, and dropped him off at the Salvation Army shelter. In college, when we girls had stayed up half the night planning our futures, I'd never been the one who was going to be counter culture. I was going to be a school teacher, for God's sake, about as middle class as you can get. Nothing prepared me to live my own life. Nothing could have.

I was frightened that Gregg would go to prison. In the nineties I'd taught a number of college courses in mostly a medium security prison for men, though once I'd worked in a maximum security facility. Given the nature of his crimes, I knew it was unlikely he'd be put in Virginia's Class D lock-up for the most violent, repeat offenders. Still, conditions in any of the long-term settings were grim. I hear people talking about how "good" criminals have it, and I'm always astonished. The total "get over, get by, get out" mentality is far more like *Law and Order* portrays it than the "you did the crime, now do the time" advocates would have us think. Yes, there are gangs in prison; yes, there are pay-offs; yes, there are drugs and serious pecking order systems. It's not hard for guards to become hardened and sadistic or jaded and on the take. It's a grim environment where most criminals become increasingly less civilized the longer they are incarcerated.

The men I worked with were the lucky ones, on Pell Grants at the time. Many were on mandatory sentences, but they knew they'd get out one day, so they had incentive to earn "good time." Plus they were bright enough and educated enough to qualify for college coursework. Even then, without any rehabilitation or transition assistance, the stories don't always end happily. I had recently testified for a former student who was on death row in an attempt to mitigate his sentence to life without parole. Men aren't always safe; that's not possible. If Gregg went in, and he wasn't on meds, I feared that any prison time would be a death sentence. He baited people, said inappropriate sexual things, made racist remarks—no way would he make it in a prison culture. I had prayed to get him home when he was missing, thinking he'd hit rock bottom. I had begged him to continue to work, to avoid becoming homeless. Now I feared there was one more black hole he could fall in, and this one could possibly be the worst.

Easter neared, and I e-mailed all of my women writer friends to hold Gregg in the light during the spring season. Many sent him cards and letters of encouragement. Salvation Army provided him a long-term bed. He was attending AA and NA meetings as required. The social worker at the jail was wonderful and compassionate. Gregg didn't resist talking to her as he had so many therapists in his past. He was frightened, too, finally. I held out hope he was "scared straight." No one else in the family did.

I picked him up by myself on the day of his hearing. He was clean. He'd cut his own hair in an attempt to look presentable. When we got to the courthouse, he ducked into the men's room to take out his nose ring without any prompting from me and gave it to me to keep. I thought, *Good grief, Charlotte, is this what it's come to? Him cutting his hair and taking out his nose ring without prompting are cause for optimism? This, from my brilliant son?* That's in fact what we had come to; I thanked Heaven for these small signs of health.

The courtroom was strange, one of those time-stopping moments. The attorney came, talked with us, and told us what to expect. The VCU guard who had arrested Gregg originally was present; so was one of the two students Gregg had solicited. The chemical analysis had come back clean, just as Gregg had testified in his deposition. Gregg's lawyer had already made an agreement with the prosecutor. She was a D.A.'s assistant, about six-three and skinny as a crane. The sentence would be five years, all served on probation: the first-year active probation, the next four pretty free. If Gregg got in any legal trouble during that time, the remaining sentence would be enforced.

I asked, "If the product was not an illegal substance, why is he getting what to me is such a stiff sentence?" Gregg's attorney explained that since he was in a drug-free school zone, even selling a substance masquerading as an illegal drug was a felony. This was the best Gregg could hope for. If the judge agreed, and he probably would, since the state was satisfied, this is what would happen.

The array of the accused was far less seamy than the earlier court. Most of these people had cleaned up. Most had on street clothes, although a few came from "in back" in prison garb. More frightening, though, was that many of those who walked in the front door went "in back" with a bailiff or deputy after they had gone before the judge. A few received fines, some got probation, but most got time. These were people who had jumped parole, broken their DUI agreements, or been found guilty of soliciting for prostitution one too many times. Gregg's attorney had quite a few cases that day. Despite her reassurance, I was nervous that Gregg would end up serving time.

He didn't. He walked out with exactly the sentence his court-appointed attorney described. He reported to his social worker, who gave him the place to call to set up his first probation appointment, and we both left the courthouse far more light-hearted than we'd entered. Imagine, we were elated he got a sentence of five years, put on probation, and was now a felon. We went to Subway for lunch and talked about his plans. Gregg was definite about continuing with the "program" and getting his life together. He didn't ever want to be homeless or to go back into jail again. Nothing could be worse than that. I had been right, he assured me; being homeless was no walk in the park. He needed to stay away from drugs, alcohol, and the street. I made him promise (this was how many times?) to stay on his meds. I understood that they robbed him of a lot in terms of dexterity and agility, but the anti-psychotics were his only window into freedom and independence. And each psychotic event exacted a price, took a mental toll that was irreversible. A peculiarity of the disease is that while intelligence remains fairly intact, judgment, social skills, and impulse control worsen. These losses are permanent. My Lord, I was thinking, *A Mexican jail, a psych ward, handcuffs, homeless on the streets, the threat of prison? What does hitting bottom mean? How much does it take? How many times?*

173

The probation officer and social worker helped Gregg fill out paperwork for disability. Everyone involved with his treatment was clear, now, that he was unable to hold down a normal, full-time job. To some, disability sounds like a free ride; for Gregg, it was an end-of-the-line terminal. The reality that he would never finish college and hold down a respectable job was a major loss. Perhaps part of his delusional thinking was that he would always "bounce back." He told me he didn't want us to visit him anymore in a group, like we had the Christmas before. It made him feel too much like the freak on display, the family failure. Of course I would respect his wishes. His "handlers" were also looking for a more permanent halfway house placement, somewhere that his medication could be supervised, and the live-in supervisor would assure he was attending his meetings. He didn't fight any of this. John was certain it was because he had no choice; if he strayed from the strict guidelines of his probation, he'd be in prison for five years. I was hopeful that within these boundaries he'd find some satisfaction and peace.

He went to coffee shops and met people to talk to, other "regulars." He worked on his play. He played guitar and found a Sunday jam that was open to all skill levels. Perhaps a year of this would enable him to experience a pattern where he could live in peace with a realistic sense of self-worth, albeit far reduced from any plans he might have had as a teenager.

He moved into a halfway house across the James in a neighborhood that was part renewed housing, part rundown. He had an elderly roommate who had been in treatment for years. Gregg said the guy stole his cigarettes. He probably did. His other roommate was young and surly. Some of the people in the house were okay, others were moody and unpredictable. One or two were downright mean or sneaky. But workers came in and cooked and cleaned. The residents had to keep their rooms orderly and follow rules, but that was about it. I gave him phone cards so we could stay in touch. He went to the library and got a Yahoo account, so we could e-mail. For the time being he was safe and sane.

I'd go into Richmond, and we'd go out for a meal or a movie or just coffee. One day, after not too many months, Gregg called and asked me to come pick him up. He was excited. When I met him, he said he'd been talking to a guy about his screenplay. The guy was a producer. He wanted it after Gregg completed his revisions. Gregg was almost sure the guy would give him a contract. This was genuine excitement, not that fake goofiness I'd seen so much over the years. He was working on handwriting his revisions. Would I re-type the whole thing for him, quickly, so he could give it to the guy? I agreed. As a writer, I didn't want to stifle his optimism, but I also wanted to temper it, to tell him that this kind of "overnight" success rarely occurs, and perhaps he should ramp down his expectations a notch or two. Who was this man? Was he sure of his credentials? Gregg was certain this guy was on the up and up. He'd checked him out, and this was certainly going to be his big break. We talked more about the play and my thoughts on needed revision, and when we parted, he was happier than I'd known him to be since he was about sixteen.

I took the screenplay home, made all of his revisions (following his dictate not to change a single word unless something was wrong in terms of spelling or grammar), and came back to Richmond to return the clean copy along with a diskette so he could make any needed adjustments himself. Gregg was still upbeat. He and the guy had met a couple of times. The man liked his ideas for another play as well. But he still didn't have an actual contract. I remained skeptical, but I didn't want to squelch Gregg's enthusiasm. For the first time in forever, he was on his medicine, making sense, looking like a "regular" person you wouldn't stare at in a crowd; perhaps a bit wild-eyed, but no more so than easily excitable people. I couldn't help thinking that if this was Gregg at his best, he could "pass." Still, I told him to proceed with caution. He asked what he could expect to get for signing, and I said, with a small press, perhaps five hundred dollars and a percentage of profits, maybe fifteen percent if he was lucky. And he should know that independents often didn't make a profit. He was affronted. That didn't sound right to him at all. He was looking for big bucks. Maybe he wouldn't "let it go" for that. Look at Matt Damon and Ben Affleck. I assured him they'd "paid their dues" and were known in the business, and besides, they had financial backing. Looking insulted, Gregg assured me he'd have to think about it. These few hours of my son near normal and optimistic stand out as moments of hope for me. I believed he might live as a satisfied person, writing, playing guitar, making friends at the coffee shop, and attending jams and AA/NA meetings. That he lived on disability was no longer a disappointment to me. That he could live a life of personal fulfillment would be a bounty.

Only that wasn't in the cards. The guy rejected Gregg's revised screenplay but assured him he'd be happy to take a look at the next one. Disappointment does not rest easy on the shoulders of people with any type of mental impairment. While Gregg continued his treatment, he became bitter and dissatisfied again. He did start work on a second screenplay, *Die A Tribe*, but not the one he'd pitched to the producer. That one would be about a farmer growing marijuana for legitimate uses for the hemp market and medical needs and exercising his civil liberties to make a living. But he wasn't ready to start it. This other one he was starting was about a young high school-age boy, Willy again, though a different Willy, trying to make his way as an "outsider" in a religious prep school. He assured me that this one would be more grounded in reality, though it did have elements of magical surrealism. Since he no longer had a computer, he was hand writing. Would I be willing to transcribe it for him when he was finished? Of course I would do that. Writing was his lifeline at the moment, and I wanted to encourage it however possible.

He met with his probation officer as ordered and continued to go to mental health and social services. The burn-outs that lived in his halfway house disturbed him. He didn't say it, but I surmised that he saw himself in them, and it was a portrait he couldn't accept. Plus anyone who had ever been there could come by any day for a meal, so he said a lot of "druggies" stopped in, one in particular who was dating one of the women residents, and that bothered him a lot. This guy always took more than his share of food. Gregg couldn't understand why they'd let a guy on drugs hang around the place. Gregg was gaining weight, too. Through all the ups and downs, he'd put on weight because of the meds, but before, he'd work it off. This time he became so "puffy" from lack of exercise, eating a carb-heavy diet, smoking, and the anti-psychotics that he could barely walk around the block without becoming out of breath. He asked if I would buy him a pair of tennis shoes so he could start to jog again, and I took him to get some that day. He hated the way he looked and felt. Gregg the athlete was gone.

Meanwhile, he searched for a new place to live on a permanent basis. A mental health facility was under construction in Richmond where each resident would have a private efficiency apartment with a living room/bedroom combo, a kitchenette, and bath. He filled out all the paperwork and received a call a few weeks later that he'd be able to move in upon completion in a month or so. This would coincide with the time period he would have to leave the halfway house. All the disability paperwork had gone through, and he was waiting for a response.

The social worker at the house had told him he probably wouldn't get full disability—the woman was sure he could work, no matter what prior professionals had determined. She hassled Gregg a bit about this, and he became edgy and defensive. He even tried washing dishes again in a restaurant, but of course he was fired. He had no transportation, he missed buses, and he was slow. I told him to ignore her; the evaluators would make the decision, not her. He did receive a check for back disability, and he used it to pay back his Nanny and Pawpie and me and John. I was thrilled by this, not at all because of the money, but because Gregg's sense of responsibility and right and wrong was reawakened. This was the biggest positive step he'd taken in years. Plus he continued to go to meetings. While he didn't select a sponsor, he was working through the steps. To my mind, he was doing everything he could.

John invited Gregg to come visit for the weekend. We called in a bus ticket for him to pick up at the Richmond counter on a spring Friday, and I met him at the Lynchburg station. For the most part, it was an amiable, quasi-relaxed visit. We cooked foods he liked, such as grilled steak and vermicelli and cheese and homemade brownies. He met our neighbors, and we went to the movies. He smoked more than either of us had realized, but he'd always go out back and sit on our patio. He drank Coca-Cola non-stop, which struck me as unhealthy, but since it was superior to drinking beer, I didn't complain. On Saturday night, Gregg and John were watching sports on television. Gregg chose that moment to tell his stepfather some "unfinished business" that he was carrying around. I knew that this was an aspect of him trying to work through some of his resentments, but he caught John off guard. He hadn't forgiven John for "kicking him out" of our home in the mountains that time for doing drugs. He couldn't understand why we had refused to let him come stay with us when he was evicted from his last living situation for not paying the rent. And why did he make Gregg pay back that money he'd borrowed since we had plenty and he was broke? I assured Gregg that I was part of all these decisions. Though I was pleased that John didn't get into an argument with Gregg, that he tried to explain why he'd made the decisions he'd made at the time, I knew that this had spoiled the visit for him.

On Sunday morning, John got up and prepared a big breakfast for the three of us, his way of saying "no hard feelings." When Gregg was slow to respond and insisted on smoking a cigarette before he sat down to eat, I could feel the tension mounting. John was certain Gregg's behavior was passive/

aggressive. I thought the medication made him particularly slow in the morning. In any case, we eventually all sat down to eat and then went to buy a few toiletries and supplies for Gregg before his bus was scheduled to leave. We hugged goodbye and told him we'd do it again, but both of us were glad when the bus pulled out, and I don't see how he could have missed our false smiles, hard as we tried to act cheerful.

Back in Richmond, Gregg waited for his disability decision, continued his AA/NA routine, and finished his second play. We found some contests, and I paid the entry fees as a sort of combined birthday/Christmas gift, since he didn't want presents at those times. He got called in to social services for some bad news, though. The new mental health facility that had accepted him—I saw his acceptance letter myself, so this wasn't a case of him misunderstanding or lying—notified him that they were withdrawing their decision. The human services person had reviewed his file, saw that he was a convicted felon, and as that was against their by-laws, he would be unable to have a place there. This was a blow. I urged Gregg to appeal the decision, giving the name of his social worker at the jail, explaining that while he was found guilty, he had not been selling drugs, he had been drug-free and in treatment for over a year, and he had no prior convictions. He did this, but his appeal was rejected. Fast on the heels of this, however, was a letter from the federal disability review board in Pennsylvania saying he had been approved for full disability, and he would receive his first check within thirty days. I hoped that this would boost him, and it seemed to at least keep him from crashing.

The problem of where to live was still unresolved. He had fulfilled all of his probation requirements except the fines. My parents had returned the money he'd repaid them as a gift, and he used part of that toward what he owed. Still, he was hundreds of dollars in debt to the city, but he could pay it when his money came through. He was still acting rationally, still "clean and sober," so I believed that since he'd gotten through his disappointment regarding his living situation, he was still on the road to recovery.

With the promise of regular income, Gregg had a safety net. He'd developed routines: library, coffee shop, meetings. Mental health would continue to provide his medication. Once he found a place to live, he should be okay. He looked for apartments on the bus line, but most were too expensive for him to pay rent and still have money for food and incidentals. He got the idea to move to Puerto Rico, and he began researching it on the internet. John talked to him and told him that was a terrible plan. Crime was rampant there. Still, Gregg looked into housing and found out that he could transfer his status and get a mental health living space. I called social services myself and found out that what he'd read was true, but they had a long waiting list, and when a room became available, it usually went to a woman with children first. Gregg would not be a priority. Some people waited years. This finally convinced him that Puerto Rico wouldn't work, so he began looking into Costa Rica. Jaison had lived there six weeks for a summer program, but he couldn't remember the name of the family he stayed with while he was learning Spanish. The more Gregg learned about Costa Rica, though, the more determined he was to move there.

His time at the halfway house ran out. He went back to a short-term shelter while he awaited his check. Turns out they'd sent it to the social service office instead of to him, so he picked up two checks and paid off his debt to the courts. Nothing was tying him to Richmond any longer.

The final blow was rejection letters from both contests. Gregg hated that; it was his real hope. An aspect of one of the competitions was a review of the work. He received considerable praise for his writing and good suggestions for what to work on in terms of a re-write. I told him that this was incredibly positive, that no writer hit pay dirt the first time out of the block, but he viewed the fact that he didn't win as a failure. This sealed his intention to go to Costa Rica.

His departure stalled because he had some banking problems, which made him furious. John and I came into town and helped him cash an income tax refund check. Someone had made a mistake on his account, and it took him days to get this straight. Finally, he was able to open a savings account where his check could be automatically deposited each month and he could get an ATM card so he could withdraw funds as he needed them. All our attempts to encourage him to stay in Virginia made no impact. Reminders of the fiascos in California and Mexico were fruitless. He wanted to get away, to start over. The cost of living was considerably less in Costa Rica. It was a peace-loving place. He had to get away from his past. He knew he'd be happy in a sunny place where no one expected him to get rich or be some successful businessman or dress preppie.

I gave up arguing. It was no use. We tried to help him make a plan for living. When he flew into the main city, San Jose, he would look up an AA/NA meeting immediately. He could go to a hostel until he scoped out a suitable living situation. There would be plenty of coffee houses. He needed to stay away from bars. At cybercafés, he could e-mail me. He had no problem with any of this. He was excited about his move and the way he'd handled the plans. He was stingy with money, so I knew that as long as he was clean he wouldn't be extravagant. But if he started drinking or using, there'd be no telling what might happen. His support system would be nil. We picked up a few belongings that he wanted us to store in our attic. He had a passport from a European trip he'd made once when he was at VCU. He considered himself set.

He called from the airport in Miami to tell me he was fine and was getting ready to board the plane for Costa Rica. He sounded happy and optimistic.

Without prompting, he told me, "I love you, Mom," and I assured him I loved him, too, and always would.

"Be safe with yourself," I directed, my all-purpose command to my children for anything they're about to do that makes me nervous. When he hung up I, felt empty and scared, but I wanted to believe he'd be okay; that after eighteen months of sobriety and medication, he was finally on the right track. I would have never chosen Costa Rica, but maybe he would make this one thing work.

CHAPTER 11 – MEXICO II, VIA COSTA RICA

Gregg did stay in touch. At first he found an inexpensive room in a house with two girls, but one had a boyfriend who made him uncomfortable, so he moved out. He started living with a sixteen-year-old prostitute. He told me she was messed up, but he loved being with her, and she loved his American-ness and his money. He left the capital city for a small provincial town nearby, and when I heard from him in late December, he was in trouble. As the result of a hustle, he'd had his backpack stolen. Everything he owned was in there, including his passport and his medicine. Left without identification or money or his psychotropic drugs, he went to the American consulate in San Jose. He said all they gave him were some McDonald's coupons. His e-mails from this period are disturbing. He asked me to send money to him through a second party, an owner of a hotel in town who had befriended him when he was stuck on the street. I e-mailed that this did not seem wise. By then, he'd determined he wanted the money sent to Western Union. I broke our house rule about giving Gregg money (food, medicine, clothing, supplies, yes; money, no) and sent him $250, the amount he requested, so he could get a bus home. During this period John and I kept Will up to date. We all worried, but had no way to do more than we were doing short of flying to Costa Rica to get him.

>*From: "Charlotte G. Morgan*

>*Subject: Hey YOU!*
>*Date: Mon, 18 Oct 2004 11:18:09 -0400*
>
>*Missin hearin from you, Gregg. Are you okay? I have waited to send a package until I hear you're where you were last - or somewhere else okay. When you wrote you were having household wars, so I've been worried. Let me know what's up, okay? I've been crazy busy. This two jobs isn't as manageable as I'd thought - four new preps, five classes, lotsa traveling. Not that I'm complaining. So what's the take on the U.S. elections in Costa Rica? Love you, Mom*

>*From: William Gregg*
>*Sent: Monday, October 18, 2004 2:09 PM*
>*To: Charlotte G. Morgan*
>*Subject: RE: Hey YOU!*

>*So mom,*

>*Im in escazu right now. I had all my belongings including my passport stolen in a gypsy hustle. It was fairly intricate. Anyway, I got picked up a day later with only the clothes on my back walking away from san jose, and they took me to*

immigration. I spent a night there in jail, then was taken to the american embassy. The american embassy gave me some mcdonalds coupons and told me to hit the streets. So, now its monday and the embassy is on holday that doesnt exist. They were insistent upon the idea that they call three family members to ask you for money. They wouldnt allow me to use the computer or the phone. Now, I heard something on the computer about emergency money and Im going to look into that, but they were frank that there was no slush fund for my emergency. Now, when i went to the embassy today to find it closed for this holiday that doesnt exist in costa rica, I told my situation to this old school virginia boy who happened by serendipitously. He has bought me a room in a bed and breakfast, and given me some cash. Do you think it would be possible for you to swing me $300 through western union til my plane flight on the third of next month. Of course, I will have seven hundred dollars deposited in my checking account at suntrust on the first of the month, but my "tarjeta" or atm/visa card was stolen as well along with my wallet. So, if you could help me right now I would appreciate it. Um here's the western union information that the embassy insisted I have after skirting the question about emergency money on several occasions.

1. Simply bring your money to any western union agent and fill out a short form.
2. Pay a service fee.
3. Get a receipt with a MONEY TRANSFER CONTROL NUMBER (MTCN) 4. iN form your receiver of the transfer 5. Your receiver can go to

*any western union agent and upon presenting
proper identification, will be paid immediately*

-G

*>From: "Charlotte M.
>Subject: RE: Hey YOU!
>Date: Mon, 18 Oct 2004 14:28:29 -0400
>
>Where do I send the money? I read
through the directions really fast, but I'm unsure
where to wire the money. Xo Mom
>*

Hey Mom,

*This nice older man from virginia is offering
me a cheaper solution for you to send money to me.
The following are the instructions to wiring money
to his bank account. So, if you haven't used western
union already, please wire any money you can send
to his account. I am asking today for help from the
embassy. If They dont help me and you cant help
me. I will be wandering the streets of san jose until
my plane returns on november 3.*

-G

*WIRE INSTRUCTIONS TO TRANSFER
AMERICAN DOLLARTO SCOTIABANK DE
COSTA RICA S.A.*

Instruct the remitting bank to send the wire transfer to:

Intermediary Bank:

Bank One International Corporation.153 West Fifty Street New York, New York 10019A.B.A. (Field 56)

Beneficiary Bank:

Scotiabank de Costa Rica S.A.Account Number: (Field 57)

Beneficiary customerAccount Number: Beneficiary Customer Name: William K(Swift field 59)

Hello Mrs. Charlotte M.,

I am the owner of the hotel where your son is staying http://casamariabedandbreakfast.com/ and I am not just an old man. I have lived in Costa Rica for 23 years and I have helped many people.
　　Yesterday my friend picked him up off the steps of the American embassy, where he was waiting. The embassy was closed yesterday.

　　My Friend gave me money for his stay for one night.
　　I have been trying to help Gregg get things together.

*He asked you to send money to my account.
It doesn't matter whether you do this.*

*I am aware of his problems. That is his need
for medication.*

*I have had 2 people in my hotel with this
problem and when they didn't have their medication
they became violent.*

*You will understand that for this reason I
am limited in my ability to continue to help your
son.*

I hope this problem doesn't happen.

Mother,

*DO NOT GO THROUGH THE EMBASSY
TO SEND ME MONEY. GO THROUGH WESTERN
UNION.*

*YOU CAN SEND THE MONEY TO ANY
WESTERN UNION IN COSTA RICA. YOU ARENT
DUMB.*

*YOU CAN FIND OUT HOW TO DO THIS. I
DONT HAVE ACCESS TO A COMPUTER AT MY
LEISURE. I HAVE NO MONEY. I HAVE ONLY
THE CLOTHES ON MY BACK. i DONT HAVE
THE ABILITY TO BE RESEARCHING HOW TO
SEND MONEY. AND ANYWAY THE DIRECTIONS
ARE SIMPLE!!!!!]*

-G

*DISREGARD THE MESSAGE ABOUT
SENDING THE MONEY TO THIS GENTLEMANS
ACCOUNT.*

THIS COUNTRY IS FUCKED UP AND I DONT TRUST ANYONE. SEND WESTERN UNION.

PRONTO.

GRACIAS

-----Original Message-----
From: Charlotte M.
Sent: Tuesday, October 19, 2004 9:33 AM
To: costarica@costarica.org
Subject: RE: Send Money william gregg

I WILL help you, but I am reluctant to send $300 to someone else's bank account -- you can understand how that sounds to me, from a distance -- like another scam. Though I am grateful this person has helped you, I have no wish to send money to his account. I have notified the embassy to notify YOU. I have told them you need help. I will continue to bird dog that from here. IF the embassy lets me know how to send money to you without identification, then I will do that. I am onto this. I will NOT let you down. I do NOT want you wandering the streets of san jose. Love, Mom

Hey mom,

I think all that I need is the MONEY TRANSFER CONTROL NUMBER (MTCN) written in the simple directions I gave you directly from the directions in the western union pamphlet. So, if that doesnt work with the piece of paper they gave me as proof of passport, then "I" will involve the embassy.

-G

>From: Charl
>To: wg
>Subject: The MTCN
>Date: Tue, 19 Oct 2004 18:01:00 EDT
>
>Okay, Gregg, I've sent $300 in cash via Western Union.
>The question is: What is your mother's maiden name? (GREGG) The MTCN is: 398-528-8544 (without the dashes).
>PLEASE do not put yourself in a position to have this ripped off; I really don't have any extra to send (took a BIG salary cut when I left the state).
>Anyway, I hope this helps you out until you can get back to Va. PLEASE let me know you're okay and that you have been able to get the money.
>I STILL think you should ask the embassy to help you get out of the country earlier. Okay? You DID contact SUNTRUST about the stolen card, didn't you?
>PLEASE let me know you've gotten this and you're okay. Love, Mom (I know you're frustrated, but it hurts my feelings when you're harsh with me via e-mail; I'm just trying to assure the money gets there safely.)

Mom,

I apologize for hurting your feelings. I have been very disillusioned in my travels in costa rica. I dont trust anyone here. I think its a very corrupt country, personally. And I admit that when the embassy treated me with disconcern, I felt, well, I have felt very desperate the past couple days. I cant describe to you the numerous ways that I have been mistreated here and I trust no one. It seems bizarre to me as well that the day I go to the embassy to check on things, an old school virginia boy just sort of happens by on a holiday that doesnt exist. Anyway thats neither here nor there.

I have contacted suntrust and cancelled my card. I will go to the embassy tomorrow and hopefully there will be a passport for me there. I WILL leave this country "muy pronto". So, that said thank you very much for being there for me as always.

I would like to speak with you this evening if you get the chance. The number where I am is:
011 (506) 528 8344

I have also left this number on your voice mail on your cellular phone.

I love you very much,
G

Will heard from him once, too, from Guatemala. Gregg explained that he needed money, probably $300, and asked his dad to send it. Will agreed to send it to the Western Union Gregg identified but assured him that it would be the last time he would ever send money to bail him out, and he need never ask again. I spoke to Gregg on the phone. He was furious, ignoring all his prior history before this event, saying he couldn't believe his dad would talk to him that way when he'd been robbed and needed help. He swore he'd never ask him for anything again. Gregg never picked up that $300 he needed to get home.

Somehow, he made his way to Mexico City to the consulate there, and he had the state department liaison he met with call me. Again, I could only feel relief that Gregg was alive and safe, though this was clearly a dreadful situation—again, in Mexico. This event could not have been more different, however, as this time he was a stranded American citizen who had been robbed, not a jailed criminal. In a day or so, I was able to call Gregg and talk to him. His voice sounded normal, though he was clearly agitated about what had happened. After our conversation, I felt I had no choice but to tell the man that Gregg was on disability, that he suffered from paranoid schizophrenia, and that he clearly needed medication. The representative was thoughtful and understanding. He'd told me all he knew at that point, though he would keep me up to date and be certain Gregg was evaluated at the hospital. I gave him Gregg's social security number so he was able to find his driver's license photo identification on the internet. This would enable him to issue Gregg a temporary passport. He gave me his own phone number and e-mail address and told me he would stay in touch with me regarding Gregg's options. After I thought for a few hours, I sent this helpful man an e-mail explaining that IF doctors were able to evaluate Gregg and provide him with medication, he could not under any circumstances take Haldol. This was a drug Gregg had had a strong allergic reaction to when he was in Eastern State Hospital. Another dose might kill him.

From: Charlotte M.
Sent: Wednesday, November 03, 2004 8:14
AM
To: costarica"costarica.org
Subject: Gregg
William L. – Could you tell me the last time
you saw/heard from Gregg? I need to notify the
embassy. I have been unable to locate him. Thank
you, Charlotte Morgan (his Mom)

Mrs. Morgan,

It was about Oct 22.

He had received $300 and he paid one night
for the room and for the telephone calls.
I ask him to leave the $50 with me to be
returned to Ben a friend of mine who brought him
here.
but he said that he had Bens email and
would return the money to him.   William L.

Prof. Morgan,
I spoke with your son on the phone about 5
minutes ago, and he gave me permission to talk to
you again. He did not give me permission to talk to
his father. I am copying my boss, Mary A., on this
message.
Based on the information you gave me as
well as my personal observations, we asked that he
be assigned to a mental facility temporarily. Doing

*so assists us in knowing how best to help him and
what sort of assistance to arrange when he returns
to the U.S. He has left the mental facility and is now
in the regular immigration holding facility again,
and we hope that he can be returned to the U.S. in
the next week or so. However, I will let you know as
the case develops and we have something more
specific. One thing which could potentially hold his
case up is that he hit an officer in the holding
facility. However, we have not been informed that
any charges are planned.*

*Gregg told me to tell you he is sane and that
he is safe for now. He wants to be deported to
Nogales, immediately south of Arizona, because
there are some members of your family in Arizona
who he would like to meet. While I understand that
you have no control over this, he also asked me to
tell you to be sure he was not put on Haldol again
as he has an allergic reaction. Finally, he said to
look in the attic for a manila folder that is in a black
knapsack which relinquishes his father's medical
power of attorney. Incidentally, if his father has a
medical power of attorney that someone can send us
it might be helpful in allowing me to speak directly
to him.*

*Here is the process from here. We are
awaiting a report from the psychiatric hospital, and
we anticipate that it will say that Gregg needs
continuing care. He would then be sent by van to
Texas and we would arrange for Catholic Social
Services to receive him. They would then place him
in an appropriate treatment facility. The other
option is that if your family and/or his insurance
has the means and the will to do so, you could buy a*

plane ticket to anywhere in the U.S. and arrange for private psychiatric assistance. In either case, anything you know about prior diagnoses or medications would be helpful.

I am sorry I have not been able to tell you more before now. Best wishes, and please contact me if I can be of further assistance.

William F
U.S. Embassy Mexico City

-----Original Message-----
From: Charlotte G.
Sent: Wednesday, November 17, 2004 9:19 AM
To: William F.
Subject: Gregg
Dear William H. -

I understand that you are limited in your ability to respond.

For your information: Once Gregg is on his medication, he becomes responsive quickly.

When he had all of his possessions stolen in Costa Rica, I understand that his medication was taken (in his backpack). This would mean that he has been without meds since the week before Oct. 22.

I hope this is helpful.

Please notify me as soon as Gregg gives permission.

I appreciate all your kindness to date.
All best, Charlotte G.

The next call I received from the state department liaison was to inform me that he could no longer talk to me, that Gregg had withdrawn his permission. As an adult, even a mentally ill adult, Gregg had the right to determine who the authorities could talk to. This man was able to tell me that prior to the date of that withdrawal that Gregg was hospitalized in their psychiatric clinic; that while this was not jail, it was secure; and he would only be able to leave when he was deemed safe and competent to travel. Medical personnel assured him that this would be in about a week. Typically, what would occur was that when an American citizen was ready to leave the country, the consulate would provide a bus ticket to a border town, in this case Laredo. He had no idea what the timeline would be for Gregg. I was appreciative of everything this man had done on my son's behalf, and told him so. After that, I had no choice but to wait and hope Gregg would contact me.

About a week later, surprisingly, the liaison called again to tell me that he had put Gregg on a bus to Laredo, and he was headed to Richmond. Before he left, Gregg had asked that he call and tell me this. He gave me the number of Catholic Charities; they had a mission to assist the homeless, and they would meet Gregg in Laredo and offer their services. It would be up to him whether he accepted or not.

> *Dr. Morgan,*
> *I presume it is "Dr." from your email address. INM has told us that they do not intend to file any charges over the altercation. While that could certainly change, we have no reason to expect that it will and hope to be able to send him home in the next week or so. We certainly have everything we need to prepare travel documentation on our end.*
> *Gregg called today and seemed extremely anxious to get out, but otherwise much calmer. I*

appreciate your note about the Haldol, and we are passing that on to INM. He repeated his desire to go to Arizona, but I don't think that is going to happen. He gave me some contact information for his bank to pay for the ticket, but I do not believe they will talk to me in his absence.

Here is what is going to happen from here. The psychiatric report we received from Mexican authorities prescribed an ongoing course of drug treatment, but says (allowing for translation from Spanish) that he is not "psychotic" and will thus not require ongoing inpatient care. That means we can not direct him to a treatment facility against his will. However, he did give us permission to talk to International Social Services (through whom we would reach Catholic Social Services, for which Gregg's religious affiliation does not matter), and we are going to arrange to have them meet Gregg at the border. They would be able to ask him what assistance he needs and try to arrange it for him. I hope we can make that happen in the next week or so.

Unfortunately, there are a couple of risks to this plan that I need to make you aware of:

1) It is possible that the person from ISS will not be able to find him when he crosses the bridge. We will coordinate with our consulate in Nuevo Laredo to avoid this, but sometimes it happens.

2) It is possible he will refuse any treatment or assistance.

I will keep you posted on what happens. I will be out of the office from Wednesday afternoon through Friday, and you may contact my colleague

Adriana Gil (copied on this email) if you have any questions during that time.

If you would like to talk to Gregg, give me a call on Tuesday. We will try to patch a call through to him and then call back and connect you. Best wishes, and I will let you know when we have more information.

William F.

-----Original Message-----
From: Charlotte G.]
Sent: Monday, November 29, 2004 10:10 AM
To: William
Subject: RE: Gregg

Thank you for your wonderful, personal update. It is such a relief to me. Please tell Gregg that we returned his backpack when he left for Costa Rica. However, I WILL look in the attic to see if there is another.

It is true: I have Gregg relatives in Tucson. I will try to get together some names in the next week. These are people I have not heard from in over 20 years (except for one aunt, who is elderly; there are young cousins, however. One is named Hans Gregg; he is in Tucson).

It is also true that Gregg has SEVERE allergic reactions to Haldol. This would indeed damage him, perhaps permanently.

The best drug I am aware of is Risperdol, but he may be aware of a newer one that he has taken which has fewer side effects.

Please give him my love. I tried to keep up with him via e-mail, but his e-mail address has been cancelled.

The Catholic Charities route would be the best at the moment. I do not want to send your entire e-mail directly to his father; instead, I will notify him that Gregg is safe and in treatment. I think that is fair.

I hope that there are no hold-ups; when Gregg does not take his medicine he is a different person. I am certain that he was in a mentally ill condition when he hit someone. If you need my statement to that effect I would be happy to provide it. He is a peace-loving young man when he is healthy.

Again, thank you. Let me know if you need anything from me.

All best, Charlotte G.

Prof. Gregg:

It looks like Gregg is going to leave tonight by van in the direction of Laredo, TX. He should arrive Wednesday morning at 9 or 10 a.m. central time. We are coordinating with the consulate in Nuevo Laredo as well as social service agencies in Laredo so that he will receive any help he is willing to receive.

You are welcomed to call or email later today if you have any questions. Please let me know how I can be of assistance.

William F.

Prof. Morgan:

Gregg is safely back in the U.S. and appears to be headed in your direction. I am sorry that things sometimes took a while and that there was a period when I could not share information with you, but I am glad that he is coming back now. Thanks for your patience, and best wishes.
And, from my old days as a college prof, best wishes with final exam week.

WF

-----Original Message-----
From: Susan O.
Sent: Thursday, December 09, 2004 2:08 PM
To: William; Wendy C(CA/OCS/ACS/WHA); Martha J(Nuevo Laredo)
Subject: RE: Gregg Our Ref: 2004-0214 - NEW DATE

Mr. Gregg arrived in Laredo and he was evaluated at the clinic. He is now on a bus headed for Richmond, VA.

*Laredo gave him the repat ER cell phone
number so he will phone if he needs assistance.*

Susan

I didn't hear from Gregg again for about six weeks. When I
did, he was in a jail in Tennessee, outside Nashville, and he was
clearly psychotic. He told me he'd been arrested for disrupting the
peace and disorderly conduct. The language he used was a distinct
indicator that he was not well. In the coarsest racist language he
told me that he was detained when the bus driver, a Black woman,
had "threatened" him and told him he'd have to leave the bus, and
all he did was "threaten" her back, saying if she touched him, he'd
throw her through the windshield. My immediate thought was that
this sounded exactly like Gregg's racial hallucinations when he
was psychotic in the Mexico airport. Since he'd been in the jail this
time, three "Brothers" had beaten him, his lip was bleeding, and
the left side of his face was numb. He wanted me to contact *Sixty
Minutes* and bring one of their journalists and a film crew down
there, because his civil rights had been violated in this "Redneck"
po-dunk town. He told me his hearing date and begged me to
arrange to be there, if I loved him at all, and to call any newspaper
reporters in the area to come right away to interview him. Then he
hit me with the worst sucker punch: While he was in Mexico,
because of me, the doctors had given him Haldol and he'd almost
choked to death on his tongue. He viewed this as my fault since I'd
told the consular rep things I had no business revealing. I was
stunned and told him I'd sent an e-mail warning the doctors there
that he was allergic to Haldol. He didn't believe me and blamed his
near-death on me. When I asked where he'd been all this time, he
laughed and said all over. He had come to Richmond but couldn't
get a room there, so he continued to roam. Eventually he'd gone
back to Mexico (how could this be?), then up into Mississippi,
where he was jailed overnight twice for being drunk and

disorderly. About nine times he'd had guns pulled on him, and I'd be pleased to know he wasn't fat anymore. He'd lost fifty pounds since he didn't have food most of this time. He was on his way back "home" when he landed in jail in Tennessee.

On this particular day, I was home alone—perhaps I was on spring break, or perhaps it was a Friday, a day I didn't work. I could hardly stand. This was all beyond bizarre. Gregg's report of his so-called "crime" was similar to what the jailer told me when I called and talked to him. He also answered yes when I asked if Gregg had been beaten by three other inmates. I requested medical attention, and he said a doctor came twice a week, and since Gregg's injuries didn't appear life-threatening, he could wait and see the doc when he came in a day or two. Also, Gregg was isolated now, and far more subdued than when he came in. I asked if he'd had any papers with him that would give us a hint as to where he'd been. The jailer said that all he had on him when he was arrested was his ATM card.

When I hung up, I went next door for my dear neighbor, Lucia, to get her to sit with me while I figured out what to do next. Lucia is as calm as I am anxious. We called John. He was teaching a studio class, but he promised to call Will to let him know Gregg's whereabouts and situation. Again I was grateful my son was alive but shaken at his condition and circumstances. I decided to call the sheriff and let him know what was going on with Gregg. I got on the internet and found the number.

The sheriff was concerned when I told him about Gregg's mental illness and need for medication. He explained, again, what had happened—in polite terms, of course, but the story was otherwise exactly what Gregg had described. I asked him to assure me that Gregg would have proper medical attention and would be out of danger while he was there. He asked me to send a fax with the information I'd given him by phone, and I hung up and did exactly that.

To: Sheriff Johnny B. &
Chief Jailer Jay R.
From: Charlotte G. Morgan
1111 Some Circle
Lynchburg, VA XXXXX
434-XXX-XXXX

Re: William Gregg Smith

Date: March 7, 2004

I understand that my son Gregg Smith is being held for disorderly conduct until his trial date March 17 at 8 a.m.

Please be aware that Gregg suffers from a debilitating mental illness and needs to be treated with anti-psychotics.

He is allergic to Haldol. If he is given Haldol he could die.

His phone call this afternoon was the first time I have heard from him since December 9, when he was given a bus ticket in Laredo, Texas. I understand that he has been wandering since that time. He tells me that he is suffering from facial numbness and a split lip due to a beating he received at the hands of four other inmates.

His father, William E. Smith, has medical power of attorney. I will try to reach him so he can be in touch with you.

Please provide Gregg with medical attention and legal advice. He is not competent to refuse either.

His father and I are very concerned for Gregg's health and safety and wish to assist in his

*legal problems and aid in his speedy return for
medical treatment.*
        Thank you for your assistance.

   I called Gregg once more and talked to him. He told me to
shut up and listen, not to interrupt. He had a letter he'd written that
he wanted to read to me. He knew I wouldn't like it, but he'd hang
up if I interrupted him. This rant was maniacal; it was in essence a
description of his "road trip" since he'd been in the hospital in
Mexico City, blaming the "redneck" law in Mississippi and
Tennessee for all his troubles and claiming he would bring lawsuits
against both states as soon as he could talk to the correct
authorities. He described in detail how he had been deprived of his
civil rights, mistreated, and harmed repeatedly at the hands of the
government and how he still wanted me to bring *Sixty Minutes* to
document all this. The language was coarse and racist. He was also
going to file suit against a particular woman at his bank who had
been stealing funds from his account. When he finished, I begged
him not to send me the letter. He insisted he was going to. I urged
him to go back on his medication, and he became furious. He
complained that I had no current information about chemistry, that
I was ignorant, that I could not imagine the side effects of those
poisons, and he would never use them again. When I suggested
that he come to Lynchburg where I would be nearby and could
help him find an apartment in a halfway house, he lost his temper.
He launched, again, into how I had never provided for him, had not
welcomed him when he was sick, had plenty of money and room
and would not let him stay with me, and just wanted to shuffle him
off to some awful living situation where he was a freak. He'd
never live in Lynchburg. He hated John, he hated his father and
older sister and brother, and if I didn't come to his trial, he'd never
see me again.

This was one of the worst conversations I'd ever had with Gregg. Maybe the worst, except for the day of his commitment hearing, which could hardly be called a conversation. I knew I couldn't drive to Tennessee and bring him back by myself, angry and psychotic as he was. It wouldn't be safe. John had to work, and he wouldn't even consider going if Gregg wasn't medicated. Gregg couldn't fly paranoid, and I certainly couldn't put him on a bus. John convinced me that if Gregg wouldn't agree to medication there was nothing I could do, so for the first time, I didn't go to his rescue. No one did. I talked to the jailer one last time before the hearing. He told me that the sheriff had called in a crisis intervention team. They'd interviewed Gregg (Remember those questions; Gregg certainly did: Are you a threat to yourself? To others? Etc.) and agreed that he was lucid and capable of understanding the charges against him. He was within his rights to refuse treatment. He had also been seen by a physician. A lawyer had been appointed, and he'd met with him. After that, neither the sheriff nor the jailer would take my calls. I suspect Gregg cut off permission for contact with me. Will called the courts and found out that Gregg had been sentenced to thirty days in jail; that's a matter of public record. He also exacted a promise from someone—the assistant to the Commonwealth's Attorney? the jailer? the sheriff? I'm not sure— that he be notified before Gregg's release.

I called Gregg once more after his trial, and he came to the phone. We talked only briefly. He blamed everything on me. He was also still angry at the woman at the bank who'd messed up his money. Money was still disappearing from his account, so he was going to confront her and make her fix it.

Before he hung up, he said, "You won't talk to me again, Mother, so this is goodbye." He waited. "Say goodbye, Mother." I didn't say anything. "Goodbye, Mother." He hung up.

That's the last time I heard his voice for so long that I came to think it might actually be goodbye. On my birthday in June,

2004, I waited all day and night to hear from him. No matter where he'd been, or what trouble he'd been in, he'd always called on my birthday. That year he didn't.

Will and I were seeing one another almost daily during this month because Melanie was ill. I had taken off from work to be with her. We talked about what to do about Gregg, and Will decided to draw up a trust with an attorney monitoring it, so Gregg could live independently. He'd be able to draw from the funds monthly, for his rent. This would enable him to live safely off the streets, with his disability money for food and expenses. Two days before his date of release, I faxed this information to the jail.

> *Gregg (Smith)*
> *S. County Jail*
> *c/o Jay R., Jailer*

> *Dear Gregg –*

> *I know you have not wanted to talk to me. Please read this letter. I will not suggest that you go into a group home.*
> *Your father is willing to make available a trust to you, for your housing costs, so you may live independently with your disability money for your own use. He would not be involved; it would be handled between you and the trust attorney (not your sister).*
> *If I could send you a bus ticket to Richmond, would you be willing to see Lisa Morris at Richmond Behavioral Health? I would find a way for you to stay in a motel until you got your apt; I would provide for food as well. None of us want you to be homeless again, ever.*

If you are unwilling to take the last medication you were taking (the one you said was not so bad?), would you at least talk to her and Richmond Behavioral Health about lithium? Early on some of your doctors suggested trying treatment for bipolar disease rather than schizophrenia. Would you consider that? I am not making that a condition of your bus ticket or motel room.

Lisa Morris refused to give your records to the judge; you can trust her, even if you believe you cannot trust me. Would you please be willing to go to see her and seek some kind of treatment that the two of you, without any say or intervention on my part, could agree on?

Your father and I understand that you do not wish to see us. I would be willing to bring whatever furniture you might need to your new apartment and leave while you unloaded it, if that would make you agreeable to the idea. He would do that, also.

I am suggesting Richmond only because your AA group and your NA group and Richmond Behavioral Health are there. If you would decide you'd rather live in Lynchburg in an apartment that is also possible.

[Personal information about his older sister, Melanie, is omitted here to protect her privacy], she said that she was ashamed of herself for the way she'd treated you.

Miranda is doing okay in college; she still has a lot of self-doubt and depression, but she's taking medication. So am I.

I am sorry that the doctors in Mexico gave you Haldol. I can show you my e-mails to the immigration officer saying that you could not take

Haldol, that it would be deadly for you. I did not
come to Tennessee because I did not see a way for
me to get you home if the judge released you, as you
sounded psychotic to me in our phone conversation.
I am sorry, but I could not do it. I guess I could
have put you on a bus and driven back myself, but I
was afraid to do that with you so angry and
spewing such hatred. I'm sure you're still angry.
I'm sorry. Please call collect (434-386-xxxx) OR
Melanie's (804-xxx-xxxx) as I may be down there
this weekend. I love you.

The jailer called me some days later, apologetic. He was so
sorry; it was clear that Gregg's father and I wanted to do what was
best for him. But he had to tell us, the judge had released Gregg
two days early. I have no way of knowing if Gregg ever received
my letter.

Deputies had driven him to the nearest town with a bus
station, gotten him a ticket, and given him enough money for food.
Aside from that, he had no idea where Gregg was.

I called the homeless shelter in that town. The man who
answered checked registration. Gregg had spent one night there.
The person I talked to had no idea where he was headed. I tried
other homeless shelters in Virginia. No one had him signing in
during that week or the next. I tried to call Richmond Mental
Health, but no one would (or legally could) return my calls. I
finally sent a fax with the information about the trust Will intended
to set up. My hope was that Gregg would come to Richmond, that
even though he was not taking any anti-psychotics, that some
limbic survival aspect of his brain would lead him back to where
he could be safe. In the cover sheet to my fax, I asked anyone who
was working with Gregg if he showed up to read my letter to him.
I called his bank to see if I could find out where he was using
ATMs; of course this is a matter of confidentiality. I knew that, but

I had to try. I couldn't remember the exact name of the woman Gregg was angry with at the bank (Jen or Jill?), but I was sure which branch he'd mentioned. No one there had a name similar to the one I vaguely recalled.

I'd followed all my trails. They all led nowhere. In the end, I couldn't find him. I would have to live with the one thing I'd always said I couldn't live with: not knowing where he was or if he was dead or alive. The thing I'd feared the most had happened. I could only pray that he'd found safety, that he wouldn't hurt himself or anyone else if he was unmedicated. Perhaps this was my sufferance, because in the end I had failed him, failed to do that one thing all mothers are supposed to do; keep her offspring safe. That was my burden, and mine alone. I am Gregg's mother.

And then, one sunny day in February, 2007...

The Letter.
That curled capital C–
cramped, disconnected letters forming
my name, my home address, in blue
ballpoint – who would write me from Montana? –
a pre-stamped envelope, some junk mail
lookalike
from Inmate # 2103246.

I know who that is.
That blink between one moment and the next,
my missing son
isn't missing any more.
This letter on my dining room table, benign
as the others, stings like scraped knees.
He's been gone three years.
"Say goodbye, Mother. This is goodbye,"
in that flat across-the-wires voice

that wasn't his
at all.

And now this envelope, this object
riveting my vision:
It's from Gregg.

I can't touch it.
                I have to touch it.

I picked it up like any piece of paper—
not hot, not cold,
only unresponsive paper.

Should I conjure some ceremony? Music? Tears?
Just squiggles on an envelope, and I cann't move. His
letter, in my hands, for me to open.

CHAPTER 12 – MONTANA

Gregg wrote a letter to me February 26, 2007. That beautiful sunny, winter afternoon when I saw his envelope from Montana on my dining room table, I thought for a moment that it had to be enchanted. What a complex instant: joy, fear, gratitude, trembling. Gregg was alive. And we'd have the chance to begin again. Much of what he wrote was incoherent. He said,

> *Hello, Mom,*
> *It feels good to be writing to you. I need your help. I have been in prison in Montana now for over a year, almost a year and a half (Please follow my handwriting, it's a "flex"-pen.) I know you don't want to be bothered with my downfalls or my homeless escapades, but I wrote a dissertation in music while I was in Billings Jail.*

Parts of the letter were illegible and incoherent, but he wrote something about being "factually the greatest guitarist and musician ever to pick up the guitar," and he did say, clearly, "So,

Mom, I have been put on Haldol . . ." I couldn't read the end of the sentence. He continued, "I need you to become political for me. My civil liberties are being denied to me. You are the only one who can help."

He signed the brief letter, "Sincerely, W. Gregg Smith (your son)."

Immediately I called the prison warden at Montana State Prison in Deer Lodge, Montana, and told him my son was incarcerated there, he was diagnosed with paranoid schizophrenia, and he was allergic to Haldol. I didn't know any details at the time—the letter didn't say why Gregg was in prison—but I didn't want him to die from an allergic reaction to Haldol like he almost did in Mexico.

When I was finally able to speak to Gregg about a week later, I heard his actual voice for the first time in years. He insisted I get a crew from *60 Minutes* to tell his story.

This started a year and a half of correspondence, talks with Gregg's psychiatrist at the hospital, getting clarity on why he was in prison, a parole hearing, and Gregg's return home on parole the late summer of 2008.

His original hearing at the Yellowstone County Courthouse on January 23, 2006, stated, "Appears to be a drifter with unresolved drug issues." His court appointed attorney, James Seligman, Esq., said, "This case did not involve use of illegal drugs, nor did it involve any drunk driving, Your Honor, nor any allegation of drunk driving, Your Honor."

Gregg had stolen a truck to "escape" to Canada. I only had every other page of the court transcript (I have no idea why every other page was retained, or why), but the pages I did have were rambling and unrelated. At one point, Gregg read from his written remarks, "According to 22-2-106, Montana Arts Council has specified duties requiring it to, one, encourage throughout the state the study and presentation of the arts and stimulate public interest and participation therein.

"Two, cooperate with public institutions, and parenthetically I've included, such as the Department of Fish, Wildlife and Parks. Engage within the state artistic and cultural activities, including—and the key words here are—but not limited to. And it goes on to arts, music, et cetera."

Incoherent? Clearly. After Gregg's rambling and unhinged discourse in his defense, the Honorable G. Todd Baugh, Thirteenth Judicial District Judge, sentenced him, "For the offense of theft, felony, the Defendant be sentenced to five years at Department of Corrections, credit for time served, restitution, $1,0021.83 as requested." Despite Gregg's obvious incoherence, neither the attorney nor the judge at any point requested a mental history or examination. Such an examination is mandatory in such a situation, but the judge did not order it.

In speaking on behalf of Gregg's parole plan in July, 2008, to the Board of Pardons, his attorney, Gregory A. Jackson, wrote, "Mr.[Smith] was seriously mentally ill at the time of his offense. He had been mentally ill (paranoid schizophrenia) for many years pre-dating the charges giving rise to his conviction in Yellowstone County. In fact, he had been deemed eligible for Social Security Disability Income (SSDI) as a result of his mental illness years prior to this offense. His long-standing mental illness is documented by the Montana State Prison Mental Health Unit's records, as well as Dr. William Stratford's report (Exhibit B).

"Remarkably, however, his mental illness was not considered at all during the course of or at the disposition of his case. This is obvious from a review of the Pre-sentence investigations report (Exhibit C), sentencing transcript (Exhibit D). There is absolutely no mention of his mental illness or his history of mental illness by his counsel, the pre-sentence author or the court. In fact, the PSR indicates 'no' psychological information— nor is there any reference to mental illness. . . Remarkably, while the sentencing transcript evidences bizarre and grandiose thinking and speech by Mr. [Smith], it is simply not commented on."

He concluded by saying, "Mr. [Smith] accepted responsibility for his actions and plead [sic] guilty. His mental illness at the time of the offense, though ignored, is beyond dispute. He is not a criminal, but rather, mentally ill. He is a bright, intelligent and promising young man."

In writing his forensic psychiatric report for the court's consideration on January 17, 2008, William D. Stratford, M.D., PC, Adult, Child, & Forensic Psychiatry, said, "Mental Health Service note from Montana State Prison on 7/12/06. 'I'm giving them something newsworthy' regarding his letters to local newspapers. He complained of his father's conspiracy to torment or kill him. 'I'm trying to prove my genius to you.' He continued, on assessment, to present with obvious signs and symptoms consistent with schizophrenia, paranoid type, after spending approximately six and a half months in isolation in the Billings County Jail. He was disorganized and delusional." [Underlinings are Doctor Stratford's.]

The justice system failed Gregg. Solitary confinement only added to his paranoia. He was not evaluated for mental illness despite his rambling remarks and other inmates refusing to be in a cell with him. He thought a guard was an evil angel harming children and that the guard attacked him. I can only imagine the outcome if he hadn't eventually written to me.

Gregg finally returned home in the late summer of 2008. Getting the local mental health system to help him was difficult. John and I went to the Community Services Board (CSB) mid-summer, tried to provide information early, and get an appointment for him the week of his release; that was impossible. They would not open a file for Gregg until he was physically present. Per their regulations, he could not pre-schedule an appointment or pre-order his medications, despite having a release date. We were well aware of the long wait time for mental health appointments at CSB, and we knew that without meds and clinical intervention, Gregg's ability to manage his return to society would be in jeopardy.

When Gregg did arrive, he only had thirty days' worth of his medication. Getting social security approval for his prescriptions obviously would take longer than that. Through even more appeals and pleading, we were finally able to get him sixty days of meds so his services could be put into place and he wouldn't have another psychotic event before he even had a chance to begin to rehabilitate.

Gregg lived with us for two months before he got his own apartment nearby. On arrival, he immediately contacted his parole officer. At Gregg's request, I went with him to his first meeting. In my presence, this man made it clear he expected Gregg to "re-offend." Gregg went to Narcotics Anonymous—ninety meetings in ninety days—and created a support group. His father came to visit every two weeks. Gregg was med compliant, drug and alcohol free. He volunteered at the Daily Bread and worked part-time for friends. He built his life again, baby step by baby step.

Gregg missed so much in those years lost to him— Miranda's college graduation, the birth of Jaison's two children, all those family holidays and beach weeks and celebrations. We lost that time with him, too.

Gregg completed community college and subsequently finished a degree in accounting at a well-respected private college in Virginia that took a chance on him. We all attended his college graduation. He was eventually employed full-time as a business manager/accountant at a company in Richmond. He went before the Virginia Board of Accounting, and they gave him permission to sit for the CPA tests. Every step of the way, he was open and honest about his history of mental illness and crime.

When Gregg first started his regimen with Abilify at the prison, after they took him off Haldol, he told me, "Mom, this is a drug, finally, I can live with."

Friends and family have sustained Gregg. In June, 2014, he was in his younger sister's wedding; Miranda and her new husband invited him to their Christmas Eve celebration in their first home.

His brother in California flew him out to become acquainted with his wife and two children. Melanie invited him to her home to look at football and basketball on TV; she asked him to house-sit for her when she traveled. He helped his niece with guitar; they talked endlessly about music. With John, he learned to cook family recipes. He confided in John and sought his advice about everything from clothes to job interviews.

Whenever he walked in the door, he hugged each of us; before he hung up the phone, he'd say "I love you." He visited his ninety-year-old grandmother often at her retirement home. He was a contributing citizen and an honorable, loving man. We were a close family, fortunate to have Gregg with us. Miranda's hopes for him, in her ethics essay, had been fulfilled.

At this point, Gregg wasn't our prodigal—he was our joy. American society by and large turns a blind eye to the serious problems and needs related to young people suffering with mental illness (particularly paranoid schizophrenia). Too often band-aids are prescribed for sucking chest wounds. Consider the disturbing rate of high school dropouts, teen suicide, adolescent violence. Many of these issues are still grounded in mental illness.

Creigh Deeds was a long-time state representative in the Virginia legislature. His son Gus was turned away at his local Bath County Hospital on November 18, 2013, because they did not have a bed for him. The next morning, he repeatedly stabbed Creigh, and then he killed himself. For want of a bed? Such loss due to unfunded mental health care is inexcusable in the richest country in the world.

Supporting one another in our fragmented way, this family never gave up, despite all the barriers along the way. I realize many stories end differently, not for lack of trying. Often it appears that the proverbial deck is stacked against the mentally ill and their families. It is. We can and should do better as a society, as a medical system, and as a legal system.

Gregg lived independently. He gave back. He could vote.

In one of his final letters from prison, on June 7, 2008, Gregg wrote, "What I'm thinking now is that: I need to do something good. I need to find new ways of spending my time constructively. I want to do good things. I want to do the right thing."

He did. What finally brought about this dramatic change? That remains enigmatic to me, much as Gregg's descent into madness does. Was it the new medication? The fear of prison? The chances he missed? Shreds of knowing he is loved getting through? The ability to be clean and sober long enough, in a controlled environment, so he could finally benefit from therapeutic help and gain control of his faculties? Aging out of the most virulent stages of the disease? The right therapist at the right moment? Some fortuitous combination of all of these? I'll never know.

CHAPTER 13 – 2018: WAY UP, WAY WAY DOWN

Each time a doctor, nurse, or technician walked into the ICU room, I jumped up and said, "Hi, I'm Gregg's mother."

From 2015 until August, 2018, I never imagined he'd be in a Medical-Surgical ICU Trauma Unit hanging on to his life by the barest thread.

Gregg met Angela on Match.com in early 2016. He was working for his father as CFO in his construction business. Angela had been on Match one day; Gregg had been on two years. They started dating, and we were thrilled when we met her that summer. She was lovely, plus a college grad, former international airline stewardess, never married, and spiritual like Gregg. When I was introduced to Angela for the first time at a local barbecue spot, I was pleased. They made eye contact, they checked in with each other if a question came up, and they leaned in. I could breathe; they were in love.

In March of 2018, Angela and Gregg eloped (with the help of his brother Jaison and Jaison's wife Molly) and were married in an Elvis Chapel in Las Vegas. From the video, Gregg was the happiest he'd been since I couldn't remember when. He whispered, "You're so beautiful," to his bride, his expression transported. Angela beamed. Molly and Jaison had tears in their eyes. This was everything I'd dared hope for since that first psychotic breakdown: Gregg was sane, healthy, in love, and loved in return.In May, Gregg came to Lynchburg for the day to see a grieving friend from his former church, and he spent a few hours visiting with John. I was out of town. That evening John told me he was worried. Gregg was pacing. And angry. And seeking John's advice because he believed that someone was embezzling at his dad's company.

Though John's radar for detecting Gregg's deviant behaviors had always been excellent, and Gregg's accusations certainly sounded paranoid, I downplayed this concern. Ten years med compliant with no incidents, college graduation, marriage. Gregg was stable. John had to be wrongheaded to be worried this time. And Gregg was over forty, a period when the power of schizophrenia diminishes for many of its sufferers who've survived that long. I assured myself Gregg was mad because his father disapproved of the Elvis Chapel marriage. Angry didn't mean paranoid. He'd get over it. Maybe someone was embezzling. Gregg could work all of this out with his dad. Not our prob. John insisted something wasn't right, that perhaps Gregg had stopped taking his meds. This once, I took a wait and see approach.

A week or so later, Gregg quit his job. He told us his dad was disrespecting him by ignoring his concerns. John called Will. Both of them thought Gregg might be off his meds. Someone needed to ask him. I drove to Richmond, and Miranda and I went to see Gregg. From the porch, we could hear him playing his guitar and singing. While he wasn't overjoyed to see us, he invited us in and relaxed somewhat as we talked. True, he was mad. True, he was pacing. But he was reasonable, assured us that he was taking his medicine, and that he was fine, looking for work. He insisted that he had to quit because his father hadn't been respectful regarding his marriage or his professional concerns. He was able to make eye contact with me. We left, uneasy but reassured that Gregg might be making bad decisions, but he wasn't psychotic.

On July 4, I was driving home early from our cabin in Bath County. The cellphone rang and I pulled off to answer it. This was odd for me. Usually I never stopped on winding Rt. 501 in the mountains. There aren't many pull offs. And I never answer my phone when I'm driving. But for some reason I did this time. It was Angela. She was weeping, having difficulty speaking.

"Gregg left me. Last night, about two in the morning. He packed his car, said he didn't love me, and left. Said he was heading west." This between sobs.

This hit me in the face like a fist. Angela assured me that Gregg WAS taking his meds. He'd just had his prescription refilled. He even took the pills with him. She'd never seen him so agitated, though—or mean. That word, "mean," jarred me.

Gregg called Angela periodically as he drove toward California. When he got there, he immediately turned around and came back to Richmond. His trip took thirteen days. When he returned, he told Angela again that he didn't love her, that he'd sleep in the spare room while he figured out what to do next, and she wasn't to talk about him with any of us. Thank goodness she kept communication open despite Gregg's irrational request.

We all conferred during this period, clear that Gregg was in some kind of schizophrenic crisis, but unclear how it had come about, with Angela's insistence that he was still on his meds. I decided that I had to see for myself, so I made up my mind to drive to Richmond after he'd been home about ten days, take Gregg to lunch, and talk to him about what was going on. He'd always talked to me in the past, except when he was psychotic. On July 20, I let Angela know my plan, and she assured me Gregg would be home. If he didn't answer the front door, the back would be unlocked and I was welcome to go in.

That July morning was hot and muggy. Typical Richmond. I parked across from Gregg's house and went up the front walk, knocked on the door. No answer. One of his kittens came to the front screen, so I petted its tummy and talked to him a minute. I decided to go around back, so I walked along the shady walkway by the side of the house toward the back fence.

Gregg jolted to the gate screaming. "Get the fuck off my property. Get out of my fuckin' yard. Who the fuck do you think you are? Get the fuck out of here!" His hair was long, greasy, and wild. He didn't have on a shirt, and his muscles bulged. He pushed through the gate, stabbed his finger at me, and shook his arm. His voice was loud and shaky with fury. I have no doubt that if he'd had a gun he would have shot me. His eyes were the worst, though. Demonic. No other word comes close.

Gregg backed me out of his yard. Every step he took forward he screamed and cursed, poking his finger inches from my face, while I moved backwards toward the sidewalk. I crossed the street and stood by my car.

He kept screaming from the porch. "Get in your fucking car. Get in your fucking car, I mean it. Get off my street. NOW."

Trembling, I drove around the corner, parked, and called the police. Talking was difficult, but I forced myself to speak, to describe Gregg's wild demeanor, his rabid threats. Two officers came. I called Crisis Intervention. I called Will. Six more policemen arrived, Will arrived, and the Crisis Team made a plan. Angela gave her permission for them to enter the house.

They searched. Gregg wasn't there. His car was still parked around the block, so he hadn't gone far. While they were figuring what to do next, Gregg strolled down the street, turned around, and offered his hands to the police to cuff, but he started screaming insults at me and his father while they walked him to a car.

"He's not my father. He's nothing to me."

Gregg was placed in Tucker Psychiatric Hospital for seventy-two hours. He'd have to appear before a magistrate. Angela talked to the liaison social worker for over an hour and gave as much of Gregg's medical and mental history as she understood. Gregg would see her but no one else.

As we waited for Gregg's hearing, John was able to dig out the key to unlock this mystery of why Gregg had relapsed. John finally asked Angela the right question and got the unfortunate but correct answer. In December or January, when Gregg went for his regular three-month med check, he saw a physician's assistant he'd never worked with before. His regular clinician was on pregnancy leave, so he had been assigned someone different. She recommended a new drug, one touted to have fewer side effects. Gregg agreed to give it a try. So he WAS taking meds, only not the Abilify that had stabilized him for ten years.

Traditional family dynamics and roles kicked in. His older sister said, "That's it. Gregg's kicked Dad in the teeth one too many times. I'm done with him. For good." His younger sister said, "Will Gregg ever lead a normal life? Is this insanity in the family? Can I get it?" His brother said, "Let me know if I need to come, if I can do anything."

Will talked to his company attorney, a wonderful, compassionate woman, and she agreed to help us through the hearing. The magistrate ordered Gregg hospitalized for up to a month at Tucker. What an odd moment: elation that my son would be ordered to undergo inpatient treatment in a psychiatric hospital. The psychiatrists there were court-ordered to get his records from his current physicians in order to get the jump on treatment.

Apparently a phone call is interpreted as a review of records, because that's all the communication that occurred between Tucker personnel and his former psychiatrist during his stay. Angela told his appointed PA at Tucker that Gregg had been healthy on Abilify, but for some reason the woman ignored Angela's input and put Gregg on Risperdal, one of the older anti-psychotics. Then they added Clozapine. And just before his three weeks there were up, they gave him a shot that would last up to a month, Invega.

Gregg doesn't remember his release from Tucker, but he went home with Angela. This is significant: He was so sick that he doesn't remember going home. The next day, he went to bed. After three days, he was so physically ill and incapacitated that Angela had to call an ambulance. Gregg was incoherent; he had no control over his bodily functions. He entered the emergency room dehydrated with a fever in excess of 106. 104 can be lethal.

Medical Diagnosis: Neuroleptic Malignant Syndrome.

I'd never heard of it. NMS. "Neuroleptic Malignant syndrome (NMS) if a life-threatening reaction that can occur in response to neuroleptic or antipsychotic medication." All three drugs, Risperdal, Clozapine, and Invega, list NMS as a risk factor, only no one ever told Gregg. Or Angela. Now he was at risk of dying.

By the time I got to the hospital, he was in MST-ICU on life support. His chance of survival was eight out of ten. The first ten days would tell. Unless his kidneys failed. If his kidneys failed, his chances went to ten to twenty percent.

Every time a doctor or a nurse or a technician came in, I stood up and said, "I'm Charlotte Morgan. I'm Gregg's mother." The connection umbilical cord-like.

A medically induced coma. Breathing tube. A cooling blanket with constant body temperature measurement. Temperature down, but previously so high it might have caused brain damage. Antibiotics. Opioids. PICC line. You name it—lines in both arms, his chest, a catheter. Pulmonologists, cardiologists, neurologists, nephrologists, urgent care specialists, everything but a psychiatrist. Medical stabilization was the primary concern.

Middle of the night, first night (a Saturday); lights dim in the room; hall lights bright, lots of activity and low noises.

Male nurse comes in with a "bag" to hang.

Me: What's in the bag?

Male nurse: Propofyl.

Me: Oh.

Male nurse turns to me, smiles: You know, the Michael Jackson drug.

Me: Oh.

Irony I note: Gregg is a recovering drug addict. The next day, when they add a bag of Fentanyl, I almost say "Oh. The PRINCE drug."

Most of the ICU nurses had never seen a case of NMS. Many of them admitted they'd barely heard of it, so everyone in that unit was rotated in and out. They were exactly what you'd pray for, smart and concerned and calm and attentive. We were assigned a nurse liaison for our questions or concerns. Even the cleaning staff were kind. One bedside radiologist was abrupt, but other than that, everyone we saw in the ICU was professional and admirable.

I hadn't brought anything with me, so my college roommate Susie picked me up and took me to Kroger to get a toothbrush and my meds. I stayed with her a couple of nights: food, wine, baseball, sleep. Then I moved in with Melanie and her family for the long haul, since doctors had no idea if/when Gregg would be able to "wake up" again. Typical: 11-14 days. Prognosis: No idea.

We set up round-the-clock family supervision for Gregg. Everyone came. Almost everyone. Both sisters took eight-hour watches. His stepmother did, too. Even his stepbrother from her side came from South Carolina to sit vigil with us for a few days. John and Will took some of the night duty, sleeping in a chair. All prior dysfunctions were history. We all feared Gregg was dying.

For this hospitalization (unlike all the other times since he'd turned eighteen), we had access to Gregg's records. Angela, as his wife, had HIPPA rights. The medical staff was open and informative and helpful and dogged—a far cry from the stand-offish, secretive, and uncooperative psychiatric staff. The Chippenham medical staff made it clear over and over: Tucker was a separate entity, a different hospital completely, despite the fact that they were both housed on the same campus.

Around the second or third morning, the young woman nurse practitioner who was Gregg's case manager while he was treated in Tucker Psychiatric came to see the family. I was ready to strangle her, and her actual physical presence did nothing to stifle that urge. She spoke faintly, acted nervous, and rarely made eye contact, even when I asked her questions. Not the type of psychiatric clinician to engender confidence or hope. The conversation did not go well.

"I'm sorry this has happened to Gregg."

"This didn't happen to him. This was done to him. He was given the wrong meds."

"The Abilify failed."

"Don't say that. Gregg was stable on Abilify for ten years. Look at him now." I nodded toward him immobile in the bed.

She cut her eyes over, back. "We followed the medical protocol."

"I don't care about your protocol. His wife told you he was successful on Abilify."

"She asked us not to give him Haldol. We didn't."

"Thank you for that. It might have killed him. But you did give him Risperdal. He told you he didn't want to take it."

"He wasn't compliant at first."

"Not wanting to take a drug he's had trouble with in the past isn't lack of compliance."

"He was surly."

"He was mentally ill, psychotic. Did you get his records?"

"I talked to his psychiatrist. He told me they'd taken Gregg off Abilify."

"Some nurse practitioner SUGGESTED a new drug. Abilify didn't fail."

This is how the conversation went. I couldn't imagine being in the hospital and having this woman manage my care. She

226

had the warmth of an ice cube and, to my mind, the diagnostic sensibility of a beagle. I refused to accept her apology.

The next morning, the acting administrator from Tucker came to see me, no doubt because I'd let our nurse liaison know that I was one hundred percent dissatisfied with the prior communication with the nurse practitioner. I'm sure her report to her boss about our conversation wasn't positive, either. This man was everything the nurse practitioner wasn't: confident, communicative, and charming. He assured me that those in charge of Gregg's care HAD received and reviewed his records, that the medical regimen was sound in his case, and that they'd followed the correct treatment plan for someone with BiPolar II.

"Bipolar II? Gregg doesn't have bipolar disorder. His diagnosis is Paranoid Schizophrenia. It has been for years."

"The treatment would be the same. And this is the diagnosis we were given from his prior psychiatrist."

"That doesn't make any sense to me. Didn't you do your own evaluation when he was admitted? And did his outside psychiatrist tell you why they took Gregg off Abilify, which stabilized him for ten years?"

"Yes. Gregg and his wife were concerned about Abilify's side effects and wanted a change."

"Gregg and his WIFE?"

"Yes."

"That doesn't make any sense. She doesn't go to his appointments with him."

He assured me that Gregg had received the best psychiatric care possible with their inpatient team at Tucker, and he was stable and ready to leave when he was discharged, after he had finally become med compliant with first the Risperdal and then the other two recommended medicines. I thanked him for his time. That was the best I could do.

This acting administrator came back to Gregg's room a couple of hours later and apologized to me. He'd "misspoken."

Twice. They had NOT requested or received written records prior to treating Gregg—just the one phone call. But he had the records now and would study them, and I could be assured that they'd done everything correctly. And oh, yes, Gregg's wife had NOT requested a med change or complained of side effects related to Abilify. That was just Gregg. Again, he apologized for "misinterpreting" his earlier review of Gregg's file.

They'd even diagnosed him wrong while he was with them: Bipolar Type II? He'd had a well-documented diagnosis of Paranoid Schizophrenia for years. This acting administrator had tried to tell me that the diagnosis didn't make that much difference, like I was some bumpkin. Later in the day when I told the neurologist, that made her flip—not a typical sight, one specialist showing disapproval of another professional's assessment. She cited misdiagnosis for mental health patients as an enormous error. Plus it had been days before we knew that Gregg had the Invega in his system, only after one of the sharp ICU nurses found it in his records. Invega is one of the drugs with a risk factor for NMS, and it would take thirty days for it to degrade in his body.

The fourth day a feeding tube, around the sixth day a machine for cleansing his kidneys, around the eighth day dialysis. The kidneys weren't working. Wait. The kidneys weren't working.

Plus sludge on the gallbladder; another tube to drain. I watched him every day and most nights as he lay inert in a coma. Physical therapists came in and worked with him, but he made no response. Docs and nurses would try to get him to press their hands, look at them, blink. It was weeks before he did either.

While Gregg was on dialysis, the doctors were able to cut back other meds gradually. On day twenty-seven, he woke. He couldn't talk, because he was still on a breathing tube, but he wrote that he wanted a Coca-Cola. I neither laughed nor cried. I was numb. He couldn't have anything to drink; he still had his breathing tube and his feeding tube.

Finally, a psychiatric physician's assistant read his records and came to interview him. What does a mentally ill person need to do to actually have a session with an actual psychiatrist these days? This young man was smart and attentive and curious and helpful. Gregg wouldn't leave the hospital until he was on an appropriate mental health regimen, but his physical health and recovery were still primary. He'd probably have to go to a rehabilitative hospital for a while. These facilities rarely have psychiatrists on staff, but they'd have one consulting. Gregg told him he wanted a Coca-Cola. At this point, Gregg had no idea he'd ever left Tucker or entered ICU, no sense of being in the hospital this time for a month.

Gregg made an unexpected, fast physical recovery once he was awake. Everyone who worked with him commented on his strength. His kidneys remained a question mark for a while, but finally he came off dialysis and went to a regular surgical room for a week before his release. As I write this on September 25, 2019, Gregg is home now. He can't go back to work yet—maybe never, full-time. He's on Abilify, and he's fine, mentally. Our family had a quiet Thanksgiving. John and I were invited to dinner with Angela, Gregg, and Angela's mom. Upbeat, we were still a bit stunned and cautious with one another. Christmas was fantastic. Gregg and Angela went with all of us on Richmond's Tacky Lights Tour, everybody hugging and laughing and enjoying the chance to be together for no reason other than fun. All old grudges were off. Melanie asked us all to her home for Christmas dinner and Tricky Santa. Gregg and Angela put together stockings for everyone. The gathering was the happiest I can remember.

Gregg is strong. He's used up lots of lives, but he continues to give us love and hope and the opportunity to understand the value of family at a cellular level. Being Gregg's mother has never been an easy path, but here we are again, fortunate to be alive.

A memory movie plays in my head: Gregg, about three, chunky, in the tiny playroom upstairs in our house on Claremont.

He has on a striped long-sleeved shirt, corduroys, and he's on the floor playing with his Weebles and his Weebles Schoolbus. He knocks the little round children over, they bounce up. His face is serious, his brow scrunched like an old man's. He's not laughing. He touches one figure with one finger, holds it down, it pops right up. I watch. This is Gregg. This is me. His mother.

APPENDIX I

1.   Excerpt, Gregg's original play, *Witch's Lament*:

1 INT: DAY

A twenty-something man shuffles through a coffee table for something.

Overview shows that he is in the middle of a living room. A long couch and a loveseat are present, but he has chosen a wooden, wicker desk chair to sit in. Eventually, through the piles of coins, magazines, textbooks, candles, he finds a guitar pick.

The lights dim, except for a spotlight which shines from the corner onto an unopened guitar case. Atop the guitar is an important cap which has the rebel flag on it.

He carefully picks a Martin guitar up out of its case after placing the hat on his head and adjusting it. The guitar cradles carefully in his lap. Spotlight completely on the man; now, there is a slow, deliberate placement of a C-chord on the fret board. He begins and finishes playing "Rose Connelly."

CUT TO:

2 INT: DIFFERENT APARTMENT; NIGHT

The sound of KNOCKING FADES IN to the scene.

KNOCK on an apartment door. The door is primarily a rectangle of glass with wooden surrounding. Four men can be seen from the inside view of the door, standing outside.

From inside the apartment, through the glass door, WILLY speaks.

WILLY:

What are you doing here, Dad?

MAN 2:

We're with Crisis Intervention. May we come into your apartment?

FATHER:

(Overlapping)

Willy, you need some help. Let us come in and talk to you.

WILLY:

Who the fuck are you? What the fuck are you doing, Dad? I'm calling the cops.

WILLY leaves the door and walks down the hall to his bedroom where he picks up the receiver of a telephone off a different coffee table in a different room. It is similar, however, in its messiness. CLOSE UP dialing 911

RECEIVER:

What is your emergency?

The four men have somehow made it into the apartment, and are standing just outside the open bedroom door, father first.

WILLY:

Yes, I have some intruders on my property. (Away from the receiver).

OUT OF MY HOUSE! (Into the receiver) One is my father, the other three I don't know, but none of 'em are welcome on my property.

RECEIVER:

Dispatch is on the way to 2405 Thomas Ave.

WILLY:

Thank you.

WILLY hangs up the phone, then he walks over to his father and shoves him. The three men turn to leave. The father turns as well. WILLY follows them up the hall.

WILLY:

GET THE FUCK OUTA MY HOUSE!! GET THE FUCK OUT NOW!!

The foursome walks out of the building and WILLY sits in the living room waiting for the police to show.

When they knock, WILLY speaks through the locked front door, making it clear that he wants no one but the two patrolmen entering his house. WILLY faces them from the fireplace in the living room. A large, circular glass table is in between them. A sofa on one side is adjacent to the fireplace, and there are corner chairs similar to the sofa.

WILLY:

I want these people removed from the premises. I'm a tenant under lease agreement . . .

COP 1:

(Overlapping)

Well, sir, apparently these Crisis Intervention people have a legally binding document called a TDO, meaning Temporary Detainment Order.

The order entitles them to legally submit you to a psychiatric facility.

WILLY:

So what does that mean? You can just come onto my property and take me off for no reason?

COP 2 holds up two black-gloved hands indicating he does not want trouble.

COP 2:

Well, it's for a reason. Apparently the doctor who issued the TDO has substantive evidence that you may be of danger to yourself or someone else, so . . .

WILLY:

But I'm on my property. I'm not hurting anybody.

COP 2 holds up his black-gloved hands again.

COP 2:

Look, we're just doing our jobs...

WILLY:

I thought your job was to keep the peace, not disrupt it. I mean, what about my constitutional rights?

COP 2:

You can make this easy, Mr. Wilson, or you can make it hard. Please don't make it the hard way.

WILLY:

This is fucking ridiculous!! I called you to get trespassers off my property, and I'm the one that gets hauled away. No fucken way.

The cops approach WILLY, after looking at one another, from either side of the table. There is a short scuffle between the three of them, and WILLY is forced to the ground with a cop's knee on the back of his neck.

INT./EXT.

WILLY is walked out of the apartment into the night and then put in the back of a well-lit paddy wagon.

2. Excerpt, *Witch's Lament*

5 INT: HOSPITAL; BEDROOM

The room is well lit. Several large male orderlies are crowded around WILLY. WILLY is cursing and fighting and being forced into submission. A nurse sticks a needle in his behind.

6 INT: HOSPITAL; LIVING AREA

WILLY:

What did you just give me, you fucking bitch?!!

NURSE:

The doctor ordered 20 mg. of Haldol. It's an anti-psychotic medication that will help you calm down.

WILLY begins having nervous twitches beginning with his arm and head. IIe cannot keep his head facing forward, and his jaw continually grits.

WILLY pounds on the Plexiglas window at the medicine station where the nurse is safely protected.

WILLY:

What the . . . fuck did you . . . just give me?

7 INT: HOSPITAL

WILLY is banging on the window of the medication room. The nurse opens the door and hands him a pamphlet. WILLY sits down to read it and grows even more irate.

WILLY:

What the . . . fuck is Tardive Dyskinesia?!!!

The nurse simply stares at WILLY through the window with a helpless look. WILLY is still twitching.

WILLY:

Can't you fucken give me something?

Nurse springs to action.

NURSE:

Here. Take this. It should take care of Haldol's side effects.

WILLY is somewhat calm now but still twitching.

WILLY:

What the fuck is it?

NURSE:

Cogentin.

8 INT: HOSPITAL

To be sure, the Central State Mental Institution Ward is mainly one large room. There are several single THIS END UP chairs and couches along with tables. The nurses' station is at the back of the room. One of the inmates sings at all times. Others sit with blank gazes. Still others have nervous twitches. A handful of the more

down to earth patients continually flirt with the nurses.

LOONEY 1:

Miss Jackson, you like to mastabate?

MS. JACKSON:

(amidst raucous laughter)

Now Jefferson, that is not funny. If you continue to make

lewd comments, I'm going to suggest that you go to the solitary

confinement room.

LOONEY 1:

Well, that's what Dr. Ebersoll like to ax me all the time. He

say, "Do you like to mastabate, Jefferson?" and then he get this

funny look on his face.

LOONEY 2:

(simultaneously, who's been singing)

Miss Jackson, can I get just a little smooch, smoochie

woochie?

LOONEY 1:

I say, 'Yeah, Dr. Ebersoll, I do like ta mastabate sometime. Not all the time, doe, cause shit just be getting messy.' And then he say, 'How often do you like to masturbate, Jefferson? Once a day? Once a week?' You know, Dr. Ebersoll, he a homo.

Looney 2 steals a peck from Miss Jackson and she chases him briefly. One of the larger inmates picks the chase up where the nurse leaves off. Looney 2 is enjoying himself, as are some of the other viewers, but most are just zombies staring into space. WILLY discontinues his laughter when he looks around. Meanwhile, Looney 1 has picked up his conversation with another nurse.

LOONEY 1:

I tell him. I says, 'I don't know, Dr. Ebersoll, sometimes I just get this feelin come over me, and I gotsta rub one out.' You understand, don't you, nurse?

LOONEY 2:

He asked me the same thing, and he asked him the same thing, too.

(They slap five, and Looney 2 begins singing) 'Say you, say me...say it for always . . .'

LOONEY 1:

Dat ain't da hand you mastabate wit, is it? (pause) Then he asks, 'How many times dat day you do it after you done it dat one time?' And I says, 'I don't know, doc, usually once is enough when it ain't the real thing.' Hey, Miss Jackson, how come you ain't interested in how often I mastabate? Seems to me like it's part of my treatment.

A tap on the shoulder rouses WILLY from his stupefied chuckle and Dr. Ebersoll, obviously a gay man, requests for WILLY to follow him.

LOONEY 2:

'Say you, say me. Say it for always. That's the way it should be.'

LOONEY 1:

(to Miss Jackson quietly).

He gonna ask that white boy all kind of funny questions.

(Loudly to WILLY)

Hey, don't let him know too much, white boy. He might just fall in love with you and keep you here forever.

The doctor walks very light in the loafers, leading WILLY to an office through another ward. Once they are in the office, the doctor sits behind the desk across from WILLY.

DOCTOR:

So, Mr. Wilson, you've been admitted here for a mental illness. My prognosis for the moment is schizophreniform –

WILLY:

I demand to get off this Haldol.

DOCTOR:

Haldol is something we administer to all patients who are in a psychotic state. Tell me, are you hearing any voices since you've been admitted to the hospital?

WILLY:

I'm not psychotic now, and I want to get off this medication. I've never been psychotic –

DOCTOR:

Denial is one of the primary symptoms of any mental illness.

WILLY:

Look, it's not illegal to hear voices. So what if I did? You can't keep me here for that, and this Haldol shit is destroying my muscular skeletal system. I'm getting twitches. I can't control my eyeballs. I keep grinding my fucken teeth.

DOCTOR:

This meeting is not about your medications. This meeting is for me to get a better idea of who you are.

WILLY:

You do know this shit can kill you, don't you?

DOCTOR:

Why do you think that you are here?

WILLY:

Because the cops put me in a paddy wagon and took me to the loony bin.

DOCTOR:

While you are here we need to understand a few things. Do you intend to be violent with the other patients?

WILLY:

Uh, no.

DOCTOR:

Do you intend to hurt yourself?

WILLY:

No.

DOCTOR:

We recognize that there is a lack of privacy at the hospital. How often do you masturbate?

WILLY:

What?! What does that have to do with anything?

DOCTOR:

Can you give me an estimated guess? Some people are required to curb their habits to respect other patients.

WILLY:

I'd say once, maybe twice a week. This place doesn't exactly turn me on.

Doctor furrows his eyebrows. He seems excited (aroused).

DOCTOR:

Well...that's not too bad. And where do you masturbate?

WILLY:

Oh my God, what do you mean?

DOCTOR:

I mean, do you masturbate in the shower, usually, or in your bed at night? Or do you occasionally masturbate by putting your hand down your pants while you are watching TV?

WILLY:

I don't see the relevance of these questions, but I'd pull my pants down and masturbate for you right now if I thought I could get out of this hellhole.

3. Excerpt, *Witch's Lament*

14 INT: APARTMENT

They enter the car and as the doors slam, the door to the apartment closes behind Father, Mother, and WILLY. The apartment is nearly empty. There is one coffee table with nothing on it. A love seat and a long sofa face the coffee table. There is one lamp at the end of the sofa. A bookshelf is also against a wall in the living room, but it holds no books. The kitchen has a 50s style Formica/fiberglass metal table with three matching chairs. The mother is very proud of this find.

MOTHER:

See that table? It's just like a 50s breakfast table. I got it with all three chairs for $20 at a yard sale.

WILLY walks down the hall and opens the bathroom door; not even a curtain on the shower. The next door to be opened is the bedroom which contains a single bed with no sheets.

FATHER:

We fixed it up as best we could considering I just signed the lease yesterday.

WILLY:

(attempting enthusiasm)

It's nice. Not quite as nice as the hospital bungalow I'm used to, but...

MOTHER:

I thought we'd go catch a matinee while we still have time, unless you had something you wanted to do with WILLY.

FATHER:

No. You two go to the movie. I've gotta be back at the office. But we do need to talk because you're going to be working with me for a while. So I'll call you in the next couple of days.

Father leaves. WILLY is very anxious and uncomfortable. He goes to the bathroom, splashes water on his face and looks at himself for a long while in the mirror.

15 INT: APT.

MOTHER:

(overly enthusiastic)

So what do you think of this apartment, huh? Pretty great,

ay Shug? I really think you're going to like it here.

WILLY:

I find it stale and boring.

MOTHER:

Don't be so cynical. Let's make a cup of tea and then we'll

sit and chat for a few minutes before the movie.

****'Golden Vanity'****

WILLY stays in the loveseat while his mother brews the tea. She is

singing an old lullaby, The Golden Vanity, in the kitchen.

WILLY:

I recognize that song.

MOTHER:

That's right. It's the one you used to love for me to sing to you when you were little.

WILLY is still dazed from the psychotropic medication.

WILLY:

I liked that song.

MOTHER:

So, what are your plans? Wake up in the morning, do some exercise, walk about the complex, play some tennis? Maybe you could start writing again. Apparently your father is going to give you some part-time work.

That should help you get into a routine. That's what you need to do is get into a routine. Then once you're settled everything will feel like normal.

WILLY:

I'll never be normal again.

MOTHER:

Don't say that, Willy. You needed to go into the hospital.

WILLY:

Maybe, maybe not. But I'll never be the same, and I'll never trust you again. Why wouldn't you just believe me, Mom? You know I wouldn't hurt anyone.

MOTHER:

Now, Willy, I know you aren't your full self, and it's going to take a while for you to come down from the Haldol the clinician gave you. So you keep taking your Cogentin.

WILLY:

Oh, you mean that stuff that blurs my vision so I can't even read?

MOTHER:

But WILLY, the doctor told you he could give you a new medication, one without all those side effects. You have an appointment with them in one month. Now, it's important to stay positive.

WILLY:

Positive? You want me to stay positive?! Look at me, Mother. What do I have to be positive about?

MOTHER:

But you have a chance to make a new start.

WILLY:

I DON'T WANT A NEW START! I WANT MY LIFE!

MY MIND! MINE! DO YOU KNOW WHAT THEY DID TO

ME IN THAT PLACE?!!

MOTHER:

You could have chosen to go to MCV Hospital.

WILLY:

WHO DOES THIS TO THEIR OWN SON?!!

WILLY'S mother is on the verge of tears, and she does not know how to handle the situation.

MOTHER:

WILLY, I know you're speaking without all of your faculties. You're on heavy sedative medication, so...

WILLY:

No, Mother, I'm perfectly lucid right now.

MOTHER:

Willy, what your father and I did, we did because we

wanted you to go to MCV.

WILLY:

They still would have given me psychotropic medications.

MOTHER:

Yes, that's correct, Willy, and the doctors, your father, and

I all agree that that's what you need to cope with your anger

caused by the voices you hear.

WILLY:

Well, I'm not hearing any voices now, Mother, but I am

angry. I just want you to leave. Leave me in my beautifully sterile

apartment.

MOTHER:

What about the movie?

WILLY:

I don't feel like it.

MOTHER:

Promise me you'll go see the county's doctor next month.

WILLY:

I'm not making any promises.

MOTHER:

Willy.

WILLY:

I'll see you later, Mom. Keep in touch.

She leaves. WILLY paces back and forth. Then he stops at his guitar and opens the cover. He picks the guitar up and sits on the loveseat, making a slow deliberate C-chord, but it sounds very dampened and wrong, and WILLY puts the guitar back down and goes into the cabinet of the bathroom and ferociously attacks the bottles of medications.

He stamps on a vial and crushes some of the pills, then goes and lies down.

4. Miranda Morgan, Narrative Essay

Miranda Morgan
May 3, 2001
Farinholt 3

April's Fool

'April is the cruelest month, breeding
Lilacs out of the dead land, mixing
Memory and desire, stirring
Dull roots with spring rain.'

-Eliot

Sunday, April 8, 2001

My only childhood memory caught on film consists of two
minutes of ancient green footage. On a spring night, tucked away
in the security and seclusion of our mountain home, my sister,
parents and I settle into our living room and press play for that
brief glimpse into the past. My sister Melanie had missed my
birthday party fifteen years earlier but, oddly enough, someone had
had a camera handy. She sits now, hunched forward in her chair, as
we wait for the fuzziness on the screen to disappear.

In a few seconds a yellowish picture is displayed full of
olive-shaded people. A little curly-topped blond toddler bobs
uncertainly across the setting, an expansive blue porch. She wears
a white dress on her undeveloped body and a determined look on
her cherub face. Birthday equals presents, one of the few things
she has detected by the newly-acquired age of two. My parents
laugh in unison as a skinny boy with tufts of rusty hair appears.
'There's the Prince,' my father exclaims, referring to my older
brother.

'That cannot be Jaison!' Melanie says, the disbelief registering on her face. Her declaration rises with each word and finally erupts in a laugh.

'Lemme see,' comes a voice from the video, bringing our attention back to the TV. The blond youngster immediately lifts two colorful plastic figurines to the hands above her. A dark-haired boy smiles, revealing teeth too large for his pre-adolescent mouth.

We stop laughing. Reality hits. My family sits staring at the screen as if we have been transported fifty years back in time and we are the first of the placid suburbanites to own a television. Melanie watches, closed-mouth, as the boy on the screen interacts with the little girl, grinning down at her. In a few seconds the picture changes. The toddler is riding in a shining, red wagon. 'It's your big brother taking you for a ride!' my mother calls from the porch, laughing and waving as the tyke is pulled by that same boy along a concrete walk lined with boxwoods. The picture goes blank. That is the end of the tape.

Saturday, April 27, 2000

As I stand at the window of my dorm room I flatten two palms on the sill and my nose against the screen. My feet move up and down, making a rat-a-tap sound on the hard, black linoleum floor. The air is thick, Richmond air. Sunshine spills into the room causing shadows from the large oak tree in front of Bacot to creep across my face. I breathe deeply, click my heels together and turn away from the window. The room is permeated with the potency of a garden full of roses from my body spray. The smell is too sweet.

The hall, usually buzzing with girls' excitement and dismay, is quiet and empty. Down on the main floor there are still no signs of life. After going to the switchboard I see where they're gathered. Standing, crammed together and chattering, is one giant, hungry organism. My entrance causes a disruption and heads turn. Their appetite is sparked.

'Hey, Miranda, where ya off to?' one of the mouths takes the first bite.

'Nowhere,' I say without hesitation. After what seems like a much-rehearsed conversation I find out they're going to Cloverfield for the class project.

'The bus is here,' one of the girls pipes, signaling their departure and my relief.

I wait a few minutes after they're gone before looking out the window again. He stands at the end of the concrete walkway, bicycle by his side. I run hastily out the entrance door to greet him. His dark curly hair hangs in shaggy pieces around his face, and he's wearing prescription black-rimmed glasses. From their appearance they could have been the same pair owned by Buddy Holly.

'Hey there, Birthday Girl,' he says, revealing a mouth full of perfect teeth. He never even had braces. 'So how does it feel to be sixteen?' he asks, while holding one hand to keep his bike balanced and the other to envelop me in an awkward hug.

'Sixteen and still can't drive,' a hurtful answer for a twenty-seven-year-old who lives without mechanized transportation. I wasn't thinking.

He asks if we can get something to eat. I rack my brain for the closest sit-down stop. After the long process of locking up his bike we stroll side-by-side through the dumpsters, parking lot, and across the street to our decided destination, Luna Grove. The heat inside is even more insufferable than the dense air outside. Small bullets of perspiration are building up around his hairline and I suggest we order at the counter and sit outside. I request a lox and bagel and diet coke, one of my new-found vices since boarding school.

The bagel is dry and the cream cheese is frozen in its aluminum packet. As I work to get it out Gregg shifts around and continues to look uncomfortably sweaty. 'Can I get you anything?

Is there a CD you want?' he asks, staring at me with sincere brown (but sometimes green) eyes.

'No, I don't really have time to listen to music,' I lie.

'Well, if you think of something you want just let me know.'

'Sure, I'll definitely think about that,' my eagerness to be agreeable coming through in my saccharine tone. My stomach tightens. I don't want any more of the bagel but I continue eating. Anything to keep my mouth preoccupied.

Once we make it back to school he asks if there is anything else we can do. No, I have a lot of things to get done. We exchange one more hug and he pedals away. I don't watch him leave and instead enter school through the side entrance.

Sunday, April 1, 2001

I'm disrupted from my sleep, a late nap starting around seven p.m., for a phone call. Sunday nights on the dorm are the best time to get calls because it's a weaning away from the weekend, a finale. I pick up the glossy black receiver on the hall phone and slowly say, 'Hello?'

'Miranda.' It's Gregg.

I gaze at one of the walls of the gray telephone booth that surrounds me. 'Hey, Gregg,' the words barely make it out of my mouth. There is a long pause.

'I guess you know,' the black receiver transmits.

I look around the booth. The glass door parallel to the bleak wall makes the hall look hazy and far away. 'Yeah, Mom talked to me about it,' I say in one breath.

'I hit rock-bottom, Miranda. I'm writing an apology letter to Nanny and Pawpie right now.'

I am confused; there are pieces of the story that I'm missing. 'Why?' I ask, regretting the question as soon as it comes from my mouth.

He sighs, pauses again, and begins his brief and bitter story. 'I was stealing from them. For drugs. I had ah . . ah coke addiction. That's why I was in the hospital. I thought you should know.'

He continues to talk and I can hear him but I'm not listening to him. The hall becomes hazier and more far away.

'... 'llo, Miranda, are you there?'

'I'm here.' I tell him something about the unconditional love of our grandparents, that they will understand. I tell him what I want to believe.

'Miranda, I love you.'

'I love you too, Gregg. Bye.' Click; the voice dies before he gets around to 'April Fools!'

I know he'll call back. I imagine he's made a check-list and he's crossing me off at that moment. I sit there for a little while, sit there and hold the dead phone. I'm April's fool.

When people began to suspect paranoid schizophrenia, my mother wouldn't believe it. He was finally diagnosed as having this disease. Mom thinks it's a shame that people can't remember what a wonderful child he was. They only know him as the socially inept, weird-looking guy. The type of person you won't leave alone with your kids.

When I found out it was easy for me to forget, especially at St. Catherine's.

Sometimes I wonder where that red wagon has gone. It's probably lost all of its shine and the wheels are certainly rusted beyond use. It will forever remain stained on my memory as it was in the video. Full of rides to come, circles around the block, waiting for spring.

5. Miranda Morgan, Ethics Research Project

Schizophrenia: A Mental Illness

Miranda Morgan

Fairman/2nd Period

February 12, 2002

Gregg _____ was born on October 1, 1972. The only difference that his mother remembers between him and her other children in the early stages of his development was the late age that he began talking. This seemed a slight anomaly because the rest of the family was quite verbal. He was active as a child, but continued to remain introverted and quiet. In school, Gregg learned to read faster than the other children. He was soon identified as a gifted student in math, and received straight A's throughout elementary and middle school. He was also a top athlete, playing football, basketball and baseball. When he reached upper school at _____ he continued to be a good student, but other aspects of his life began to change. He began to complain that certain teachers were cruel to him. He would make inappropriate comments in class. He also began to drink heavily. At age 16 he was found passed out at a stoplight at Malvern and Monument; the car engine cut off. His parents took him to a psychologist who identified that he had a problem with anger. More drinking and lashing out incidences occurred. The summer after his junior year Gregg was placed against his will in an adolescent treatment program for one month. By the end of that time he had been diagnosed with alcohol abuse and depression. An educational specialist assisted his family in finding a place more suitable for Gregg to finish his high-school career. The desired school was one that could handle Gregg's intelligence and his problems. One was located in Maine but during that interview Gregg was hostile and refused to cooperate. He was not accepted at the prospective school. Still, he was taken out of _____ and put in a more restrictive environment for his senior year. His parents thought perhaps clearer boundaries would help. He only rebelled more. The first event that signaled that his problems were worse than had been diagnosed occurred during football season. He ran away from the team bus and his coach. His therapist was baffled. His lack of cooperation increasingly became worse. He was continually late for school, confrontational with teachers and hostile with authority. Still his grades were good and his S.A.T.'s superior. He was accepted into JMU but was asked not to attend his own [high school] graduation. The family was hopeful that Gregg would thrive in a college atmosphere but, inevitably, he did not. After failing numerous classes he was finally kicked out for pulling a fire alarm. He blamed the school. His accusations quickly turned to friends and loved ones.

After going through countless doctors and diagnoses, it has been established that my brother, Gregg _____, has a disease called schizophrenia. Schizophrenia is a mind-altering disorder that causes hallucinations and delusions. It has been called "one of the most disabling and emotionally devastating illnesses known to man." It is a brain disease that inhibits the mind from distinguishing fantasy from reality. In this essay I am going to discuss the symptoms, misconceptions, forms, causes, medications, moral dilemmas and personal affects that are associated with this horrible disease that has plagued my brother and millions like him.

Although there are many symptoms that indicate some form of personality disorder, there are a few signs that are common exclusively to schizophrenia. People with this disease suffer delusions, hallucinations, negative behavior, chaotic and jumbled thinking and catatonia. Delusions are fixed beliefs and perceptions that are true to the person with schizophrenia, but are not real.

Often delusions are paranoid thoughts and suspicions. In Gregg's delusional states he would often complain that people in our family were "out to get him." The schizophrenia would also cause him to hallucinate. While he was away from home he would regularly call my parents at night and tell them he could hear people whispering about him in the next room. This is a common symptom of schizophrenia. The hallucinations are not always auditory. Many times they are in the form of visions, smells or feelings. One example I found was of a person who felt like insects were crawling beneath his skin. This is a tactile hallucination. Negative behavior is another symptom of the disease. The phrase "negative behavior" encompasses everything from social isolation to reduced hygiene. This behavior includes showing an inappropriate display of emotion, such as laughter during a funeral, or lacking in emotion completely. This emotional deficiency is termed "flat affect" or catatonia when discussing schizophrenia. Being in a catatonic state a person is not able to move a certain area of his or her body, or communicate with others.

The varied symptoms of schizophrenia often lead other people to have misconceptions about this disease. Schizophrenia is not one disorder, but rather a group of similar characteristics. Because delusions and hallucinations are two parts of schizophrenia many people often confuse this disorder with split personality disorder. The two are in no way related. The prefix "schizo" is a Greek derivation meaning "split" or "split from the mind." This word "refers to the way schizophrenics are split from reality."

There are three main types of schizophrenia: Disorganized Schizophrenia, Catatonic Schizophrenia, and Paranoid Schizophrenia. Although this disease is broken into different branches, a victim can suffer the symptoms of all three. Disorganized Schizophrenia describes people who have trouble organizing their speech and thought. They often show little to no emotion. Catatonic Schizophrenia is when the person loses the abiltity to move. I interviewed psychologist Debra Smyth who gave an account of one woman with Catatonic schizophrenia. Dr. Smyth told me that the woman could not interact or respond to her environment in any way. She was eventually moved to a state hospital. During her entire time with Dr. Smyth she never came out of this catatonic condition. The last form is Paranoid Schizophrenia, and it is the one I most often associate with Gregg. "Paranoid Schizophrenia" is the term given when delusions and hallucinations are most prevalent in the disease.

Schizophrenia is a biological disease. People with schizophrenia are genetically predisposed. One of the hardest factors to handle about this disorder is that it does not usually show up until late adolescence or early adulthood. For men, schizophrenia is most dominant from ages 16 - 25. Gregg's major deterioration began at 16 and at age 24 he was diagnosed as schizophrenic. Women usually show signs of schizophrenia later than men, starting around 20 - 30 years old. Because this disease changes a person later in life, often in families parents feel a sense of guilt that they have done something wrong to cause the disease. I remember how hard it was for my parents to accept that Gregg has schizophrenia. They wondered if they could've done something to prevent his horrible episodes. They have come to understand, as most families do, that nature, not nurture, is the cause of schizophrenia.

Oddly schizophrenia is one of the most prevalent of mental illnesses. About 1 out of every 100 people in the United States suffer from some form of schizophrenia. This is equivalent to about 1% of the population.

Medication and treatment for schizophrenia has come a long way in the past decade. While there is no cure, many people live successful and productive lives by taking antipsychotic medication. These drugs often cause the patient to lose feeling or response in certain muscles or areas of the body. I often felt like Gregg's medication turned him into a zombie. When he takes his medication he is not able to do some things well such as play the guitar. Gregg is a talented musician, but the medication hinders his ability to play with the talent he truly possesses because his response time is significantly slowed down.

I asked Dr. Smyth if any one case of schizophrenia stood out in her mind. She answered that one did. One woman was admitted to a hospital because she had stopped taking her medication and was suffering severe delusions and psychosis. When the woman was in a calm state Dr. Smyth asked her if she remembered anything about her irrational episodes. The woman said that they were the most terrifying experiences of her life. She was living in a perpetual hell.

The moral dilemma associated with schizophrenia arises with the issue of money. A large number of the homeless have some form of mental disease, making it the government's responsibility to provide them with health care. An estimated 32.5 billion dollars per year in the United States goes towards care for those diagnosed with schizophrenia alone. I know the personal toll schizophrenia has on people suffering from it, and on their families. In Gregg's case my family is able to provide the financial means to support him and his disease. Even so, the past few years have been physically and emotionally draining for those involved in his treatment. I cannot imagine what it would be like if my family were not able to offer Gregg medication and care. From my perspective I think the government has a moral responsibility to help the mentally ill who cannot help themselves. Thankfully Gregg has a support system; some people diagnosed with schizophrenia do not, in large part because they alienate everyone they encounter.

My entire family has worked hard to love and help Gregg, but schizophrenia is a horror that seems to negate any of our efforts. My mother makes a conscious effort to say, "Gregg has schizophrenia," instead of, "Gregg is a schizophrenic," because she doesn't want the disease to define him, but in a way it does. His newer medication is amazing compared to the older drugs, but still, they don't give him back any kind of natural ease, social grace, or physical poise. My family prays he takes his medication and stays clean, but it's a sad, lonely life, even treated. We take each step with him, but we don't live inside his head. It must be awful. Off medication he's tormented; on medication he feels half himself. There are successful, productive people who suffer from schizophrenia, but his psychiatrist tells us that even so, many continue a pattern of going off the medication. We can only hope that he can be one of the ones who finds the strength and love to stay in his treatment program and find some measure of success, though it in no way fulfills the promise he once showed as a child. For him, finishing college and leading a life of safety, independence, and sanity would be success enough.

APPENDIX II
2006 AUTHOR ANALYSIS, WRITTEN WHILE GREGG WAS MISSING: LOOKING BACK, LOOKING AHEAD

As I write this, I wait for Gregg to call me, to tell me he is alive. The last call was over a year ago, in 2004, from a jail in Tennessee, when he refused to take his medicine ever again and told me "Say goodbye, Mother. This is goodbye."

Friends have asked, "Did writing this book about you and Gregg give you a sense of catharsis?" The question surprises me. If they mean releasing emotions that I have kept pent up or hidden, the answer has to be no. I have made no secret of Gregg's problems from my first understanding of them. My birth family were secret keepers. I had no idea my maternal grandfather was alive until he died, when I was in my thirties. We children had always been told he was dead. The truth was, he was a severe alcoholic, and my grandmother sent him away when her three daughters were teenagers, saying from then on he was dead to them. They were sworn to secrecy. I've seen first-hand how damaging dishonesty can be to family openness and interaction. Now I describe my feelings, and I try to tell the truth, not to cause others pain, but to give them the gifts of knowledge and honesty. Unfortunately, these can hurt. That's the paradox.

Others have asked, "Did telling Gregg's story, and yours, give you a sense of closure?" That, too, befuddles me. I can't imagine a mother ever having closure over damage or loss of her child. I've always been a nervous Nelly, and from the time my first daughter was born I've feared for the health and safety of each child every day. I'm the Mom who'd keep the bassinet by her bed for weeks, one hand on the baby at night, to be certain she was breathing. Nothing, not any degree of fear or grief or anger, could diminish my love for my four children or make me wish they'd never been born. They've all made me laugh and made me cry, and at times confused and unhinged me. While it is true that Gregg has undoubtedly given me the most heartache, that in no way absolves me of a shred of mother love for him. Love for a child isn't about fairness or parity. I've told each of them that one of the mysteries of a mother's heart is that it stretches to love each child completely. Perhaps one day I will come to a level of acceptance of the life Gregg and I have lived together, but never closure. Love doesn't close. Some memories don't fade.

One insensitivity to mental illness that does make me bristle involves my response to language people use when they're talking about those who suffer from mental disease. When I hear people say so-and-so "is schizophrenic," I cringe. I cannot say Gregg is a paranoid schizophrenic, as though that defines him. He has paranoid schizophrenia or suffers from that mental illness. That is not all he is now or all he ever was. He is a human being with a horrible disease, and to define him exclusively by that disease is uninformed and unfair. The people who use the term "schizo" as slang for kind of goofy or out of it disturb me, also, just as those who use inappropriate physical, racial, sexual, or ethnic slurs. Simply put, that's unkind and cruel and oftentimes ignorant.

As I've researched paranoid schizophrenia all this knowledge has helped my understanding, though not resolved anything. I'm glad to know that the reproduction rate in people with schizophrenia is far lower than in the rest of the population. That's a comfort, as though nature is trying to correct a horrible design mistake. I wasn't seeking resolution as I wrote, though. I didn't even know at the time what resolution would look like. Magic, I suspect: Gregg coming home, research discovering better medication, him on the medication finding his way to a productive, happy life.

And age has taught me to go forward, not to play coulda, woulda, shoulda, and not to expect catharsis or closure or resolution, or to find some single thing to point a finger at and say aha, that would have changed Gregg's life and kept him whole and healthy and sane. Perhaps he was never whole and healthy, or, closer to reality, perhaps he was whole and healthy for sixteen years, and we who love him should count our blessings for that.

Still, as I've written this memoir troubling questions have risen to the surface. Most of them are questions I've asked myself a thousand times in the past. Some I'll never be able to answer, even knowing more facts and more information about the circumstances.

Of course, the first question that haunts me is the remark that my obstetrician made on my last prenatal exam. Was Gregg a child who didn't want to be born? That sounds so psycho-babble, but a writer friend from California assures me that this is quite likely. I'm not a devotee of pseudo-psychology or new age spiritualism. I am a reader, a fact gatherer, but still I am a layman where medicine is concerned. It does appear undoubted, though, that something was wrong with Gregg's in utero experience. I had severe flu when I was expecting him. Could this have caused a brain wrinkle at some critical point of his development? Research tells us little about the causation of schizophrenia, other than that it is a genetic marker of sorts, and it usually follows the male line.

There's tons of mental illness in my family, but not paranoid schizophrenia. I prefer to see his illness like creation: it started somewhere, but where remains a mystery.

In recent years, I have looked up post-term birth and have been astonished by what science has to say about the dangers of this condition. If I should be guilty and self-critical for anything, it's for remaining mute while I carried Gregg an extra month. In the early seventies, the mother was too often the patient, not the advocate. My daughters and daughter-in-law are assertive about any and all medical treatment. Today it's clear that any pregnancy beyond 42 weeks is post-term. A pregnancy in this stage with accompanying growth stagnation or reversal increases the risk of stillbirth. As the placenta "ages," its nutrient richness declines. Amniotic fluid may decrease. Overall, the environment for the fetus isn't as healthy, period. It was only at that last visit, after the 24-hour urine collection and analysis that the o.b. even considered that the baby might be post-term. Even then, he waited for delivery to begin normally. Science today is far superior, in terms of determining fetal age; cranial measurement is accurate within days.

The more I have learned about the trauma of Gregg's actual labor and delivery, the more aware I have become of the consequences of my passivity. I was dilated six plus centimeters upon arrival at the hospital, and the baby hadn't begun to turn or get his head in the right position, and my first delivery had taken only six hours. O.B.s do deliveries every day; they are well aware of the statistics and probabilities, and each birth is different. I never brought up the potential need for a Caesarian, never asked the indicators or the risks. The baby was small, but he was post-term, he was "sunny side up," and he didn't budge after the doctor manually ruptured the membranes. I ask myself why I agreed to Pitocin (synthetic oxytocin)? It only caused the contractions to increase, meaning the baby was pushing his head harder against an opening that wouldn't open. Couldn't that cause head trauma? If I was told of the potential side effects at the hospital, I was alone, I was not rational enough to make the decision, and the possible consequences to the baby were not elaborated. Probably my biggest misjudgment, and the one that is most easily resolved for others, was not insisting someone stay in the room with me at all times. During times of stress most of us aren't capable of making decisions rationally. I certainly wasn't.

And forceps? This is a common current description of forceps—so common it's unattributed public domain: "Forceps are instruments that are placed on the baby's head to turn the baby and/or assist the mother with delivery. Forceps are most commonly used when the baby is in the lower portion of the vaginal outlet (low forceps delivery). Only on rare occasions would forceps be applied in a higher position. If forceps marks (small reddened areas on the baby's cheeks) appear, they tend to disappear quickly." (The italics are not mine.) I gave the doctor permission to use them, but what did I know at the time? Gregg did not have "reddened areas" on his "cheeks." He had dark bruises on his temples.

I described Gregg's birth to a female friend who is an experienced anesthesiologist. For the first time I understood the two "versions" of forceps that I remembered so clearly from the delivery room. This is what my friend told me: The forceps are typically used to make an opening so the baby can slide out more easily. They should never be used to drag a baby from the womb. My doctor friend added, "Sounds to me like Gregg should have had a Caesarian delivery."

Do I think Gregg had head trauma during his labor and delivery? I certainly do. Could this have any relation at all to his later mental illness? Impossible to say. As I look backward at the information, it's troubling. The cause of Gregg's neonatal jaundice was never determined, but inducing labor has this condition as a potential side effect. Pitocin is one form of inducing labor. While my labor had begun naturally, albeit late, the Pitocin made it increase, with no increased presentation of the baby through the birth canal.

Blaming the doctor is an easy out for every medical problem these days, but I do not suggest there was any medical error or causative connection for Gregg's mental problems. Still, I would be foolish not to consider the possibility that this cluster of maternal/medical decisions surrounding his in utero and birth experiences might have been contributing, even if they were not causative.

Much of the research related to schizophrenia indicates that while the genetic predisposition is inborn, triggering events "awaken" the likelihood of active disease. What I am saying here is that if doctors had explained the dangers of post-term, mal-presentation, Pitocin, and forceps, I might have been able to make more informed decisions. His due date was September 3rd; he was born October 1st. While C-section is not without risks, there is no doubt that in Gregg's case his head and blood supply would have been less jeopardized. I can't go back and change the facts, so I would alert any woman dealing with any of these medical decisions to pay careful attention to the risk factors. Gather information. I would want my daughters and daughter-in-law to have full knowledge of any delivery options while they have time to study, reflect, and make clear though difficult choices.

Certainly, there are some decisions that had an impact on Gregg that were within my knowledge and control. My divorce was one. Gregg's father is an honorable man; I have never said otherwise. I remain certain, however, that I married too young, was not a mature wife to him, and the continuation of our marriage would not have been healthy for any of the four of us. Will is remarried to a woman who's stood by him. Melanie is a beautiful, successful woman with a precious daughter, many close friends, and a professional career. As a grown person, she understands my need to divorce when she was young, though she still bears the scars. Gregg was clearly the most hurt, and there's no excuse for that, nor do I offer any. That's on me. But in all honesty, I've never read any study that says divorce has any relationship to paranoid schizophrenia. Did I cause my children pain and anger? Without a doubt. Did I love them as much as is humanly possible, and do my best in terms of raising them in a blended family? I am sure of that. I wish I'd done something, anything, when that pre-school teacher's aide said that Gregg was angry. That was a missed moment when I might have made a difference. My sins are on my shoulders, and I live with that, but I will not wallow in my mistakes. They are part of my past. I choose to go forward, every day, loving each of my children as the individuals they are, hoping for Gregg to achieve happiness.

In doing that, I have made space for each of the other three to come to his or her own decisions regarding Gregg and their relationship to him. Schizophrenia and the toll it exacts on the sufferer often blows families apart. The anger and confusion and frustration as we each try to come to grips with the changes and losses in Gregg's life, the unpredictable behaviors, and the impact on us, can be relentless. With each crisis, new wounds open, and old jagged ones are poked and inflamed. If there is one thing I have tried to prevent, it is the break-up of this family because of Gregg's mental illness. When he is actively ill, Gregg gives nothing back; that is part of the disease. But we don't have to agree on how we feel or deal with it, and we don't. Each of the children has handled the adult relationship with him differently, and I have never tried to get Melanie or Jaison or Miranda to bend to my wishes regarding him. One is mostly estranged from him and has been for some time; one has tried hard to understand and stay in touch but, even before his disappearance, has gone long periods without contact because of Gregg's inappropriate, hurtful comments; and one loves Gregg unconditionally but experiences worry and pain being around him or even discussing him. I do not try to push my ideas on them or force them to understand my feelings or actions. I do what I have to do, and I never interfere with their choices as they do the same. I believe that each one loves Gregg in his or her heart, but for each that love is different. So be it.

Some things were within Gregg's control before the fragile thread of sanity snapped, and he threw many opportunities away while he still had the ability to make sane choices. He blew his chances in private school, when he had the option to start over. He was so stubborn with his therapists that he derailed those chances for realistic early help. He turned to drugs and alcohol over and over and over to deaden his pain. He refused to try when he was in the adolescent treatment center, when he could've stayed on meds, when he was clean and on meds but quit AA or NA, when he left the country instead of staying and having the courage to face his problems.

Things outside my control, that made me angry at the time, only make me sad now. All of us lost our tempers with Gregg at one time or another—most parents do that at some point—but I will never understand how any adult could have been mean to him, or belittled him, or bullied him, especially a family member. That's downright cruel: inexcusable and unforgivable. I wish one teacher or therapist or coach had gotten through to him at some point when he was a teenager. More often than not, adolescents will listen to other adults they respect before they'll listen to parents. I wish the school in Maine had accepted him; they could have made a difference. I wish he'd made the basketball team that one last time; he deserved a chance. Or he'd gotten his screenplay published. And so very much later, that the new mental health residential facility that accepted him could have let him move in: He'd been on his meds over a year, he was off probation, he wasn't a danger or a violent person. Not then.

The quality of care for the severely mentally ill in this rich, modern country is shameful. Once as I sat waiting for hours for help for my child, who was becoming increasingly irrational as we anticipated the arrival of a crisis team (that would ask the same questions I've memorized, and Gregg's memorized), I had an emergency room nurse tell me, "I would never work in a hospital on the psychiatric ward." When I asked "Why?" she responded,

"Because the in-patient treatment is more insane than the patients."
Only the chronically ill who have entered extended psychosis stay
"in." The others are turned out on the street as soon as they're
"cleared" by two psychiatrists (remember those questions?), even
if that means they're homeless. Only half of the approximately two
million Americans with paranoid schizophrenia are in a hospital or
institution at this moment. The others are at home or living
independently or on the street. Once they're over 18, they're in the
driver's seat, no matter how many times they've been hospitalized
(unless they actually do something harmful to themselves or
someone else—and then it's too late). They cannot be made to take
medication or attend treatment programs. We require more
managed care of our dogs.

Patients with paranoid schizophrenia learn to be sly, to say
whatever it takes to stay out of the hospital. They commit
voluntarily because they know they can get out in 48 or 72 hours.
They lie because the voices tell them to lie. And the system knows
this and lets it happen because it's "legal." Immoral? Yes.
Unethical? You bet. But still legal by today's standards. You see
the results every time you travel to a city and go to a library or
coffee shop or public park.

In the end, I have no way of knowing that anything I did or
said, that anything Gregg did or said, that anything anyone did or
said would have made any difference. Perhaps even if all of the
circumstances had played out in an ideal way, he would have still
become mentally ill. In fact, that's the likelihood. So while looking
back gives me clarity, it does not make me hard on myself or him.
Paranoid schizophrenia is a mean, mysterious disease. Stranger
still, twenty-five percent of those diagnosed will recover within ten
years, whether they're on medications regularly or not. Gregg was
not one of those "lucky" ones. I have wondered, at times, if the
descriptions of demonic possession in the Bible actually portray
ancient people with mental illness. Paranoid schizophrenia robs
intelligent, sensitive human beings of judgment, of impulse

control, of social awareness, of compassion, of empathy, of any care for any other human. It leaves the shell of the person walking and talking, not even looking like the person they were before.

Many of the medications are almost as bad as the disease. While they enable the sufferer to function, the "drug cocktail" often doesn't let him function as the person he was, or could have been. Most young people go off the meds because they hate the limited, peculiar person they become when they take them. They never feel "right," because they aren't. Other people are naturally uncomfortable around those suffering with paranoid schizophrenia, as though some reverse pheromone is sending out a warning signal: watch out, these people are weird.

These days television shows often portray those with paranoid schizophrenia as violent, though the incidence of violence to others is quite low in the overall population. They hurt themselves. They are the homeless people on the street talking to themselves. Their grooming is poor. Their nutrition is poor. They have no friends, not even animals. They are incapable of caring for anyone or anything. They are cut off from family. They hoard their few odd belongings in garbage bags and shopping carts. They survive, but that is all.

One of them is Gregg, my once-beautiful son who won his elementary school's spelling bee when he was in third grade, who sang "Hush Little Baby" to his sister, who hit grand slam home runs, earned Presidential Awards in Physical Fitness AND Academic Fitness, who could play classical guitar, who has spent periods of his life ill and alone and lost. It's not his fault. It's not my fault. It just is.

APPENDIX III
RESOURCES

SARDAA: Schizophrenia and Related Disorders and Alliance of America, www.sardaa.org/

Schizophrenia - American Psychological Association, apa.org/topics/schiz/index.aspx

Schizophrenia | psychiatry.org - American Psychiatric **Association**, www.psychiatry.org/**schizophrenia**

Support Groups:

Schizophrenia.com: **schizophrenia**.com/coping.html

National Alliance for the Mentally Ill - NAMI: www.nami.org/

Bring Change 2 Mind: bringchange2mind.org/

A Beautiful Mind by Sylvia Nasar (and the movie by the same name)

Angelhead: My Brother's Descent into Madness by Greg Bottoms

POSTSCRIPT

I am the mother of an adult son who suffers from paranoid schizophrenia. From Gregg's traumatic birth to his turbulent childhood, through his troubled teens up to the present, I have loved him, though at times that has been in the inscrutable dark. Each mother's story is different. My story, as Gregg's mother, is unique, but in some aspect all mothers will find in our intertwined lives an aspect of their own. "Not me," one might say, "that could never happen to me and my child"—and in that thought itself we are alike.

Even as the events I write about occurred, I could not believe some of the horrors I faced with this boy of mine. Scarier than any movie, more fear-filled than any imagined boogie-man, our experiences have brought me to my knees, put me flat on my back, and threatened to blow apart our family in ways no mythic monster could. Yet I survive, wife and mother of three other beloved children. My wishes for Gregg are simple now, quite different from the college and professional future we foresaw when he was young. I want him to be safe, to be healthy, to find some measure of happiness, to shut up the whispering voices and shut out the hallucinations.

"Coulda, woulda, shoulda: these are wasted words," I've said often to my husband and children. Instead of what might have been, in a bad or sad situation, I encourage us all to look ahead, to how we can solve similar problems in the future. How can we use an experience to do things differently next time? Nowhere do I need to accept my own advice more willingly than in my life with Gregg. As I write this, I don't have the luxury of predicting what next, though I hope for "an angle of repose" daily. The last time things were smooth lasted ten years.

But looking back has value, too. Sometimes, given distance, a person can understand her relationships better by reviewing things that have happened between her and her loved ones. Or, by reflecting on how she's handled situations in the past, she may get a stronger sense of who she is now. Or examination may lead to acceptance, even of those things we at first deem too defeating to bear, those matters we push into the nether-mind places and resolve to forget. Science revealed recently that a fetus' in utero cells migrate in the mother and can live inside her up to forty years; I know Gregg lives inside me. Since I could never forget him or "write him off" or out of my life, I must reflect.

I write this now because I have to. I write this to look back, to paint a mother-son portrait, to say to anyone with a troubled child that this is what we did, this is our truth. I do not attempt to say shoulda, woulda, coulda to myself or others. I do not try to assign blame to myself or others either, or to justify my behaviors or advocate some maternal philosophy. I strive to tell our story in all its messy honesty. Every memory is filtered, though, through the mind of the person describing it. If certain moments are telescoped and others are disorganized, that is the flaw of my recollection. Without hesitation, I can say that each event that I relate happened. Might I have something out of order here or there? Of course. I'm not checking records, though I have searched for real names of real people who helped us. These are my realities as I remember them. Any other person would have a different story to tell, because they didn't experience any moment the way I did, from my vantage as Gregg's mother.

Maybe by putting Gregg's life on the page I'll come to a level of acceptance I haven't yet reached. Maybe in reading about him, someone else will gain a deeper understanding of a troubled person in his or her life or burrow down for one more shred of compassion when she encounters "one of the funny ones" on the street or in a coffeeshop. Maybe some reader will get angry and try to do something to improve the mental health services and legal constraints in her town or city or state. Each person's story matters.

I have chosen to write this true story without seeking permission from anyone. I want to be clear: This is my story, as Gregg's mother. I am willing to speak for myself, only, because I do not have the right to speak for anyone else. Roshoman: Any of the other people involved would have a different vantage, a different story. For that reason, I have used my real name, because I want to be as truthful and open as humanly possible. For that reason, also, I have not used others' "real" or full name, except for professionals who were helpful. My mother's family name, Smith, is the name I have chosen as a cover for others. I have decided to "protect the innocent" as well as the guilty, because this is a book about a mother and her son and the lives they shared. Others participated in many ways, but they may not want their stories told.

I wrote the original memoir in 2006 while Gregg was still missing. The account of his imprisonment and return in 2008 are essential. The problems in our legal system, dealing with the mentally ill, and the barriers in our mental health support systems are aspects of our experience that need to be told. And the 2018 episodes: Treatment by some mental health personnel can add to the problems rather than aid in the remedy. These are my actual experiences. Gregg has given his blessing for me to publish them. Any way they can illuminate the journey through mental health problems and traumas for anyone else is well worth the pain of describing them.

ABOUT THE AUTHOR

Charlotte Gregg Morgan grew up in the "Christ-haunted South" of Richmond, Virginia, where religion dictated more than uplifted, and a portion of the population was hung up in the past while others were struggling to find freedom, fairness, and a way forward into the future. Sin and guilt and judgment were a way of life. Her excellent public schooling introduced her to the possibilities, opportunities, complexities, and diversity of contemporary life.

Morgan's first novel, *One August Day*, was nominated for the annual fiction award by the Library of Virginia. *Protecting Elvis* is available on Amazon or at Barnes & Noble. Kirkus Review (Oct. 19, 2016) called the novel "A subtle, affecting glimpse into the lives of a trio of singular women molded by the works and personal character of a rock icon." *The Family* chronicles a young woman's search for faith, family, and friendship. Who can Eileena Clayton trust as she navigates belonging and romance and finding her way in a troubled world?

Finishing Line Press published her chapbook, *Time Travel,* in the summer of 2020.

One of Morgan's short stories is included in *The Pushcart Prize Collection XXIV*. She holds an MFA from Virginia Commonwealth University, where she studied with famed author Lee Smith and "Macarthur Genius" Paule Marshall.

Morgan's fiction explores the lives of women, their compelling inner conflicts as they face the demanding struggles of complicated external lives, and the difficulty forming and sustaining independence.

She enjoys teaching adults, doing readings, and speaking with book groups and is available for workshops and presentations.

Morgan is writer-in-residence each summer at Nimrod Hall Summer Arts Program where she works with writers in all stages of their careers. Her four adult children are individual and varied and independent in their lives and careers. She lives in Lynchburg, Virginia, with her artist husband John Dure Morgan and two sassy standard poodles.

www.ingramcontent.com/pod-product-compliance
Lightning Source LLC
Chambersburg PA
CBHW020247030426
42336CB00010B/661